Schroth Therapy

Hans-Rudolf Weiss
Christa Lehnert-Schroth
Marc Moramarco

Schroth Therapy

Advancements in Conservative Scoliosis Treatment

Hans-Rudolf Weiss

Impressum / Imprint
Bibliografische Information der Deutschen Nationalbibliothek: Die Deutsche Nationalbibliothek verzeichnet diese Publikation in der Deutschen Nationalbibliografie; detaillierte bibliografische Daten sind im Internet über http://dnb.d-nb.de abrufbar.
Alle in diesem Buch genannten Marken und Produktnamen unterliegen warenzeichen-, marken- oder patentrechtlichem Schutz bzw. sind Warenzeichen oder eingetragene Warenzeichen der jeweiligen Inhaber. Die Wiedergabe von Marken, Produktnamen, Gebrauchsnamen, Handelsnamen, Warenbezeichnungen u.s.w. in diesem Werk berechtigt auch ohne besondere Kennzeichnung nicht zu der Annahme, dass solche Namen im Sinne der Warenzeichen- und Markenschutzgesetzgebung als frei zu betrachten wären und daher von jedermann benutzt werden dürften.

Bibliographic information published by the Deutsche Nationalbibliothek: The Deutsche Nationalbibliothek lists this publication in the Deutsche Nationalbibliografie; detailed bibliographic data are available in the Internet at http://dnb.d-nb.de.
Any brand names and product names mentioned in this book are subject to trademark, brand or patent protection and are trademarks or registered trademarks of their respective holders. The use of brand names, product names, common names, trade names, product descriptions etc. even without a particular marking in this work is in no way to be construed to mean that such names may be regarded as unrestricted in respect of trademark and brand protection legislation and could thus be used by anyone.

Coverbild / Cover image: www.ingimage.com

Verlag / Publisher:
LAP LAMBERT Academic Publishing
ist ein Imprint der / is a trademark of
OmniScriptum GmbH & Co. KG
Heinrich-Böcking-Str. 6-8, 66121 Saarbrücken, Deutschland / Germany
Email: info@lap-publishing.com

Herstellung: siehe letzte Seite /
Printed at: see last page
ISBN: 978-3-659-66795-4

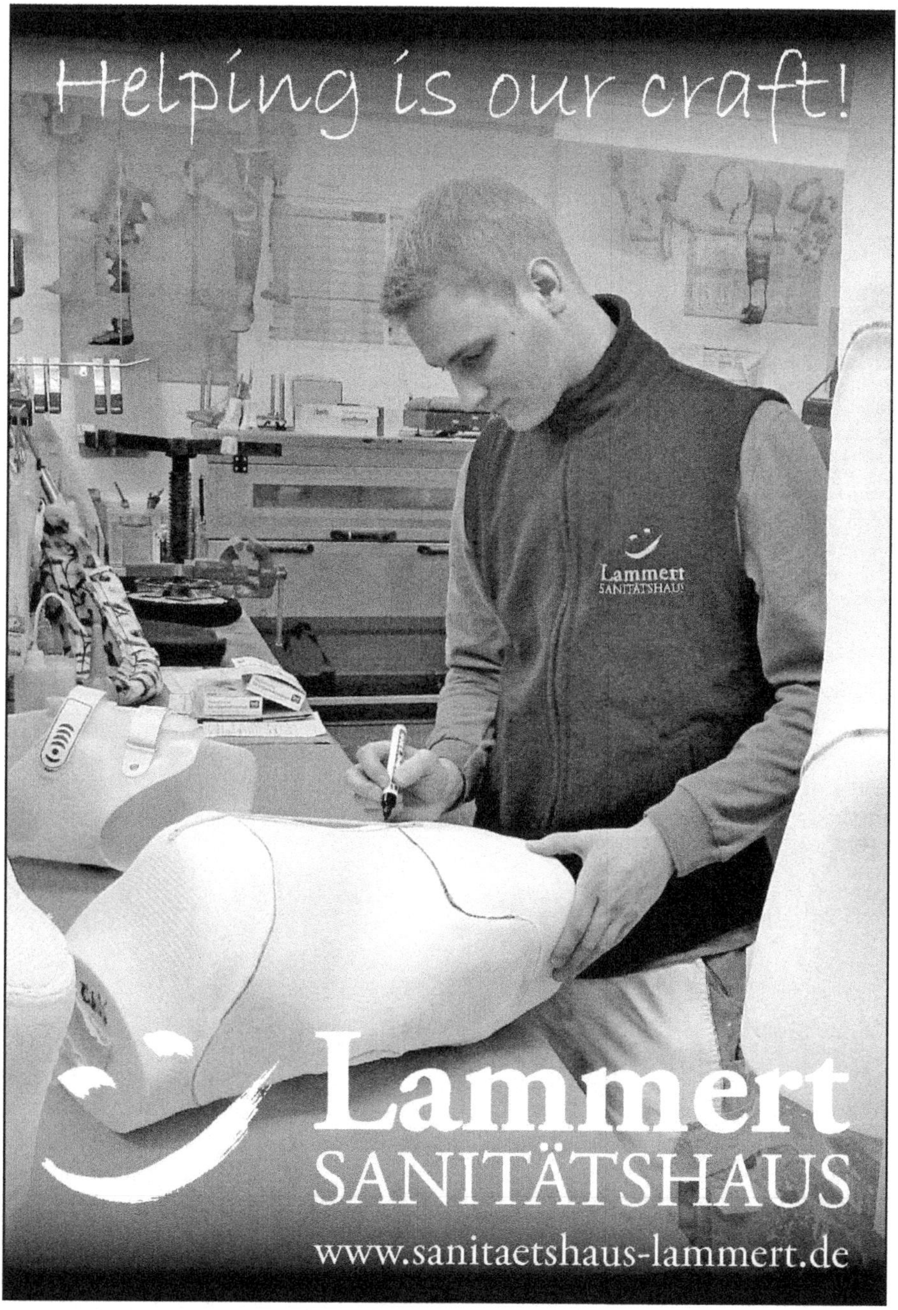
Helping is our craft!
Lammert
SANITÄTSHAUS
Lammert
SANITÄTSHAUS
www.sanitaetshaus-lammert.de

ORIGINAL-ATMUNGS-ORTHOPÄDIE
SCHROTH / MEISSEN, BOSELWEG 02

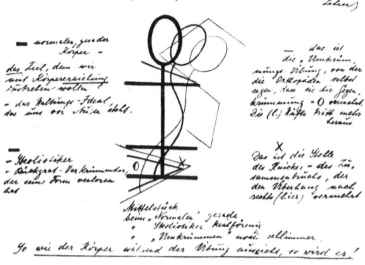

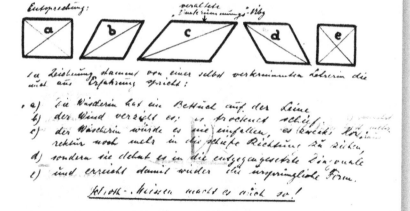

Original manuscript by Katharina Schroth

Schroth Therapy

Advancements in Conservative Scoliosis Treatment

A completely revised and expanded text about the newest
Schroth practices, based on the 3rd edition of the German
'Befundgerechte Physiotherapie bei Skoliose', Pflaum, Munich

Authors:

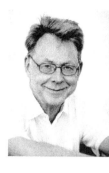

Dr. Hans-Rudolf Weiss

Orthopedic Surgeon, Physical Medicine and Rehabilitation
Specialist, Chiropractor
Gesundheitsforum Nahetal
Alzeyer Str. 23
D-55457 Gensingen, Germany
Tel.: ++49 (0)67 27 89 40 40 Fax: ++49 (0)67 27 89 40 429
hr.weiss@skoliose-dr-weiss.com
www.scoliosis-dr-weiss.com

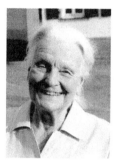

Christa Lehnert-Schroth, P.T.

Physiotherapist
Staudernheimer Straße 60
D-55566 Bad Sobernheim, Germany
www.schroth-skoliosebehandlung.de

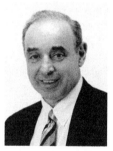

Dr. Marc Moramarco

Chiropractor, Schroth Method Certified, Schroth Best-Practice
Advanced Instructor
3 Baldwin Green Common
Suite 204
Woburn, MA 01801
781-938-8558
info@scoliosis3dc.com
www.scoliosis3dc.com

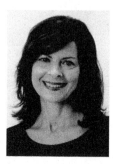

With participation of:

Kathryn Moramarco

3 Baldwin Green Common
Suite 204
Woburn, MA 01801
781-938-8558
info@scoliosis3dc.com
www.scoliosis3dc.com

Foreword

It was with great joy that I set about editing the book *Physiotherapy Specific to Scoliosis* once the third edition was sold out. Looking through the book, it was quickly apparent that by no means could it still be considered up to date in its existing form.

Having been completely re-worked in 2011, *Physiotherapy Specific to Scoliosis* was expanded further. The history of Katharina Schroth's three-dimensional scoliosis treatment was added as a sub-chapter to the history of conservative scoliosis treatments.

The physio-logic® program, addressing scoliosis in the sagittal plane, has been left more or less in its original form since presented in the 3rd edition. Physio-logic® is followed by instruction in everyday activities specific to an individual's scoliotic spine, and the exercises from the program "3D made easy," which were developed out of these everyday activities. This group of exercises should always be considered a forerunner to the Schroth program, and indeed patients will understand the somewhat more complex original Schroth exercises much more quickly and easily after having previously learned exercises from the "3D made easy" program.

The 3rd edition includes further developments of the Schroth concept from the "New Power Schroth" or "Schroth Best Practice" program as we call it today. These exercises are most suitable for mild to moderate scoliosis and severe lumbar scoliosis. With these exercises, the discussion is restricted to the most critical, those exercises in the upright starting position.

To my chagrin, I have become aware that elsewhere Schroth exercises are carried out with the patient often in a lying position, being instructed by more or less educated therapists who crawl around the patient to provide appropriate tactile stimuli.

It is only when standing or in an upright position that the patient can activate the appropriate postural reflexes. These reflexes provide an automatic basis correction before the execution of the exercise from which the actual exercise is "grafted." In contrast, when starting in a lying position, certain powerful and invigorating mechanisms cannot be accessed.

There is one argument that is repeatedly made in favor of a lying or horizontal position: that the secondary curvature can be better kept in check. I disagree, and regard it as an art to control the secondary curvature while in an upright position, an art in danger of disappearing.

Generally, we know that correction focus is principally concerned with the major curvature. Now that it is recognized that double curvatures remain the most stable after cessation of growth – as well as being the least conspicuous – I have introduced the following paradigm: if, approaching the end of growth, it is no longer possible to recompensate sufficiently for a decompensated curvature when concerned with a secondary curvature, one may indeed accept an increase in the secondary curvature if this leads to a recompensation of the primary curvature and therefore, of the entire trunk.

For a thoracic curvature with a Cobb angle of more than 70° (increasingly rare), the original Schroth exercises are still the most suitable. With these curvatures, rotation is usually so pronounced that only an antikyphotic exercise approach can help. In the case of some lesser curves with flatback, or mild to moderate scoliosis, antikyphotic exercise may not be prudent. These original Schroth exercises that promote antikyphotic correction have not yet been considered in my book. For this reason the editions up to and including the third were not yet complete.

I am exceptionally pleased to have gained my mother, Christa Lehnert-Schroth, as a coauthor of this work. She proofed the third edition of the book and contributed a chapter about the exercises from Katharina Schroth's program that were originally developed for severe thoracic curvatures. I am eternally grateful!

I am also grateful for the contributions of my friend and colleague, Dr. Marc Moramarco. He is the Chêneau-Gensingen® brace provider in the U.S. and an advanced Best Practice instructor whose passion and commitment to conservative scoliosis treatment is unsurpassed. He has provided a new chapter which adds valuable insights for the practitioner as well as help make this edition clear and more user friendly in English.

Kathryn Moramarco contributed so much to copyediting and improvement of this book that she deserves very special thanks for her untiring support.

Now that similar results in international outpatient centers treating youth scoliosis patients are comparable to the results from the unique inpatient circumstances in Germany, inpatient rehabilitation with treatment lasting several weeks has suffered a loss of esteem. Intensive outpatient concepts will undoubtedly experience an upturn in the future when one takes the effort, costs, and results of an inpatient versus outpatient setting into consideration. Therefore, in this edition, I have removed a chapter previously dedicated to inpatient rehabilitation.

Certain adult patients with scoliosis may require an inpatient environment for rehabilitation in cases of functional impairment and chronic pain, as well as a period of several weeks removed from their social environment in order to have a secure space for specific exercises to master the necessary coping strategies. Others however, experience success in an outpatient setting.

The chapter on brace provision has been tailored to the current state of knowledge and now also contains a description of scoliosis braces that meet the Best Practice standard: braces that excel at correction and are more easily wearable. Here we will also debunk 'myths' that continue to mislead people affected by scoliosis. This chapter has been taken out of the scoliosis guide written for patients and has remained largely unchanged (this book is also available from LAP). We emphatically believe that practitioners who regularly treat scoliosis patients should have a basic knowledge of bracing protocols and also the radiology of scoliosis in order to provide the most comprehensive advice.

This book is intended to serve as a foundation for a new and easily comprehensible system of instructional courses for physiotherapists and doctors. With the assistance of the techniques described here, it is possible for physiotherapists and doctors to treat patients with minor curvatures of less than 30° after a one weekend course (A level). For those with patients with curvatures exceeding 30°, we offer an advanced course (B level).

I am very grateful to Mrs. Eva Neureuther from Pflaum Press (Pflaum Verlag) for her continuous support. I am also very happy to have received the copyright for the English translation of this book. With it, I am now able to satisfy the significant international interest and provide insight into the methods of contemporary conservative scoliosis treatment, as well as provide international instructors a book to accompany their course work.

I would like to thank Mr. Patric Dressel for the creation and editing of the more up-to-date images for the original Schroth Program, which appear for the first time in this edition. Thanks also go to Mrs. Ferdinand for her friendly support.

In this new edition, several images of patients in exercise situations are included for the first time. These patients and their parents have very kindly given me their permission for these images. Thanks to Tiyen, her mother Vivien, and her aunt Elaine. Thanks also to Nicole, Kristina, and Alexandra ('Sasha'), as well as to the many other patients who had already appeared in the third edition.

My daughters Anna and Paula deserve particular thanks. They patiently stood as models for many of the exercises in this book and were thus an enormous help to me.

I must also say a huge thank you to my mother for her willingness to become a coauthor of this new edition and, in doing so, to bring this book to completeness.

I am indeed eternally thankful to Kathryn and Dr. Marc Moramarco for their great help, copyediting (so many times) and contributions making this book a unique and comprehensive textbook for therapists and patients as well.

Many thanks also to all the readers who have made this new edition necessary.

Gensingen, January, 2015, Hans-Rudolf Weiss

Contents:

1 Introduction

In the past, scoliosis was defined as a partially structural lateral distortion of the spine, meaning that the spine could no longer be straightened out completely (Heine and Meister 1972, Meister 1980, Asher and Burton 2006, Weiss and Moramarco 2013). In contrast to the types of scoliosis with a known etiology (hereditary scoliosis, neurogenic scoliosis, myogenic scoliosis, scoliosis due to metabolic diseases or systemic diseases), idiopathic scoliosis (Fig. 1.1) appears without visible cause before the attainment of skeletal maturity (Heine 1980, Perdriolle and Vidal 1985, Weiss and Moramarco 2013).

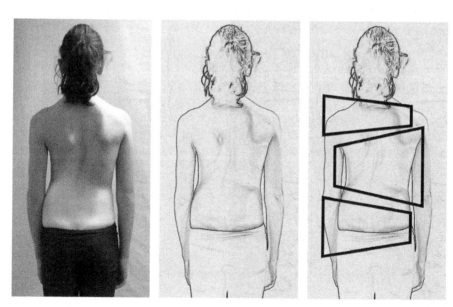

Fig. 1.1: Clearly visible scoliosis in a 13-year-old patient. All scoliosis traits are clearly identifiable: (1) deviation from the vertical, (2) costal hump as an expression of the twisting of the trunk sections against each other, and (3) flat-back with clear reduction of the kyphosis in the thoracic spinal section. In the middle image, the lateral deviation of the spine is clearly visible, and on the right, one can see how the trunk sections have pushed against each other.

Idiopathic scoliosis accounts for 80-90% of all cases. An asymmetrical silhouette of the trunk, when standing, can be taken as evidence of a scoliosis. It is in the forward-bending test where the structural component of the scoliosis can be seen most clearly. This is due to the costal hump or lumbar bulge that appears in this position. In addition, a "ventral costal hump" evolves due to the ribs on the thoracic concave side being twisted in a ventral direction.

The diagnosis of scoliosis is verified by an x-ray of the entire spine in a standing position (Fig. 1.2).

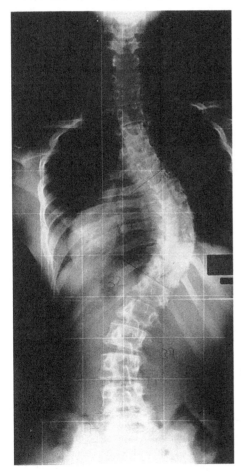

Fig. 1.2: Full-spine image in a standing position. In digital x-ray, through direct radiography (DR), the necessary region (Region of Interest/ROI) for children and adolescents can now almost always fit onto a DR plate using optimal settings.

In the age of digital x-ray, one can optimize the settings in the processing in such a way that a small image is sufficient, thus reducing the exposure time (one-plate technique, Weiss and Seibel 2013, Fig. 1.3). For patients with a height greater than 170 cm, however, it is usually necessary to make two partial images and join them together.

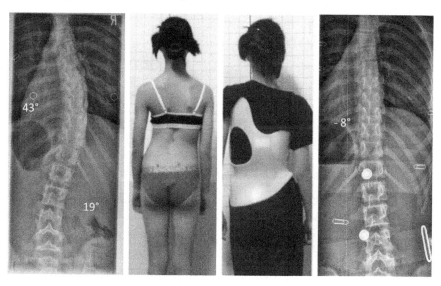

Fig. 1.3: In digital x-ray, through direct radiography (DR), the necessary region (Region of Interest/ROI) for children and adolescents can now almost always fit onto a DR plate using optimal settings. In doing so, exposure to radiation outside the ROI is eliminated. Left, patient without brace clinically and radiographically with a 43° curve; right, patient in the brace with full correction of the curvature. Reduction of the diagnostic field did not reduce the necessary information on either x-ray.

Assessment of the x-ray images consists of measuring the degree of curvature using Cobb's method (1948, Fig. 1.4), measuring the rotation of the apical vertebra, and examining the osseous signs of maturity (Fig. 1.5). Curvatures of less than 10° are not defined as scoliosis by Cobb (1948).

Females are roughly four times more likely to be affected by idiopathic scoliosis. The frequency of curvatures of less than 10° is the same for males as for females; however, the more marked the curvature is, the greater the proportion of sufferers that are females (Weinstein 1985 and 1986, Asher and Burton 2006).

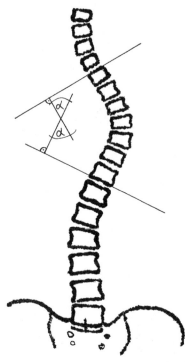

Fig. 1.4: Schematic representation of the curvature angle formation. The plate covering the upper end vertebra, which generally is tilted the most, has been marked with a tangent line, as has the end plate of the lower end vertebra. Vertical lines (on the left side of the image here) are aligned with these tangents, crossing to form the curvature angle according to Cobb (labeled here with the angle symbol).

We do not yet have reliable information regarding the natural course of untreated idiopathic scoliosis. In recent literature, there have been varied observations regarding progression, particularly since the conditions in the individual studies differed by sample. The concept 'progression' has also been defined in different ways. However, it is possible that minor spinal distortions may resolve (Brooks et al 1975, Rogala et al 1978, Asher and Burton 2006). In contrast, Sahlstrand and Lidstrom (1980) and Lonstein and Carlson (1984) agree that curvatures of greater dimensions, in statistical terms, lead to progression far more often. With a comparable curvature, females are four to ten times more likely to experience progression than males, depending on the Cobb angle (Weinstein 1985, Asher and Burton 2006). As skeletal maturity increases, the risk of progression decreases, although with more severe curvatures a significant tendency towards deterioration can exist despite skeletal maturity.

Upon reaching skeletal maturity, the tendency towards increased curvature is markedly lower. Duriez (1967), Collis and Ponseti (1969), and Weinstein

(1986) discovered that a curvature can, in principle, increase over a lifetime. However, this typically only affects curvatures of 30° or more, with the most seriously affected cases being between 50° and 75° at the point of skeletal maturity. These curvatures will continue to increase by 0.5-1° per year (Weinstein, 1986). Caillens et al. (1991) report that in the case of major lumbar scoliosis, for people between the ages of 50 and 70, an annual progression of more than 2° can occur. Within this study, an increase of curvature of more than 5° per year in patients between the ages of 65 and 80 was possible. However, it is not yet clear whether these increases in curvature are of medical significance.

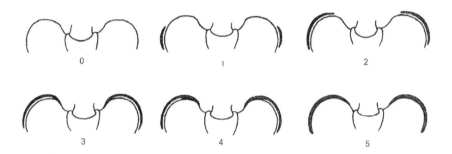

Fig. 1.5: Representation of bone maturity according to Risser in the style of Henke (1982). The Risser sign refers to the amount of calcification of the iliac crest of the human pelvis as a measure of maturity. With a Risser 0, the pubertal growth spurt is yet to happen or just happening (when the first signs of maturation are visible); from a Risser value of 3, the pubertal growth spurt is nearly complete. A fully completed growth spurt is shown by a Risser value of 5, although in some cases, a Risser value of 4 will remain into adulthood.

The main aim of rehabilitative efforts is, therefore, preventing increases in curvature (stabilization), as well as the preservation or improvement of functionality. Secondary goals include the prevention of subsequent functional disruptions, which can manifest themselves either in terms of the musculoskeletal system or cardiopulmonary system.

The study carried out by Collis and Ponseti (1969) showed that people suffering from scoliosis were no more affected by back pain than a control group not suffering from scoliosis. In later studies (Weiss 1993a, Weiss et al. 1999, Asher and Burton 2006), no connection between the degree of curvature and back pain could be correlated. It is interesting to note that

15

inasmuch as pain is present, patients with scoliosis experience a higher susceptibility to pain in the area of the curvature's apex (Weiss 1993a). Even though there is no correlation between the degree of curvature and pain in patients suffering from scoliosis, pain can be reduced effectively with intensive physiotherapy (Weiss 1993a, Weiss et al. 1999).

Generally, patients with scoliosis are concerned with constrictions in the cardiopulmonary region. However, in most cases, these fears are unfounded. According to Pehrsson et al. (1992), after completion of growth, curvatures of less than 100° do not lead to cardiopulmonary constrictions that would reduce life expectancy. Patients with curvatures of less than 100° after completion of growth are, therefore, not threatened by cor pulmonale. On the other hand, there is no indication that those afflicted with curvatures of significantly more than 100° cannot live to the age of eighty, nor will they necessarily suffer from a lower quality of life. What is known, however, is that impairments of the breathing apparatus, and performance in general, can exist even in cases of very slight curvatures (DiRocco and Vaccaro 1988, Weber et al. 1975). For this reason, the rehabilitation of breathing plays a role in physiotherapy for scoliosis, not only to correct the scoliotic breathing pattern, but also for improving breathing function and, thereby, the general performance of those affected.

The physiotherapeutic and gymnastic treatment of scoliosis has a long tradition in Europe and particularly in Germany. In Europe, there are a multitude of specialized centers that concern themselves with physiotherapy for patients with scoliosis. For twenty years, there was a European society for the physiotherapeutic treatment of scoliosis (Groupe Européen Kinésithérapie Travail sur la Scoliose, GEKTS) whose members exchanged information and ideas on an annual basis at academic congresses for the advancement of physiotherapeutic approaches. This group is now part of the organization SIRER (Société Internationale de Recherches et d'Etudes sur le Rachis), although the treatment of scoliosis has remained a strong focus. Due to language barriers, there has been a limited amount of contact between this originally French-speaking society and German- or English-speaking specialists. Today, there is the international society SOSORT (Society of Scoliosis Orthopaedic and Rehabilitation Treatment), of which Weiss and Moramarco are founding members. SOSORT was established to improve the standards of conservative treatment on an international level, but surgeons are playing a greater role with each passing year and the focus seems to have shifted somewhat.

Over the years, in Germany, there have been a variety of physiotherapeutic approaches used for treatment. Those that ultimately established themselves were the techniques based on developmental-kinesiologic foundations (Vojta and E-technique [E-Technik]) for early treatment of scoliosis, and Katharina Schroth's three-dimensional scoliosis treatment.

The PEP technique (peripherally evoked posture reaction) described in this book is also used today for early treatment, predominantly with children under the age of ten.

New findings concerning the potential of scoliosis to be corrected (van Loon et al. 2008) determined that the lateral distortion of the spine and the spinal rotation can be minimized with a simple corrective movement. Simply by increasing the lumbar lordosis at the height of the second lumbar vertebra in association with an increase of the kyphosis in the lower ribcage area, a decline in the lateral distortion is possible. Consequently, recently more exercises concerning the correction of the sagittal profile are being integrated into the Schroth concept. These physio-logic® exercises have visibly improved the results of treatment, when incorporated into patient rehabilitation (Weiss and Klein 2006).

The long-term prognosis for adolescent idiopathic scoliosis (AIS) is, on the whole, favorable. However, the signs and symptoms of idiopathic scoliosis are of importance, even when present to a minor degree (Hawes and O'Brien 2006). These cases must have target parameters of conservative scoliosis treatment due to their economic significance such as increased susceptibility or the inability to work.

In the long-term, scoliosis sufferers who have had brace treatment or have been operated upon can expect increased deterioration and, according to contemporary studies, a slightly higher level of pain, versus a control group without scoliosis (Danielson and Nachemson 2001; Danielsson, Viklund, Pehrsson and Nachemson 2001). Also, in the long-term, impairments due to scoliosis are the same for patients regardless if they have had surgery or not. Therefore, impairments (loss of function, reduction in general health, increase in pain, and impairment in lung function) cannot be precluded by undergoing surgery. Recent Cochrane Reviews from Romano et al. (2012) and Negrini et al. (2010) have shown that both physiotherapy for scoliosis and brace provision count as evidence-based methods of treatment. In this context, it is interesting to mention the randomized, controlled study from China according to which non-specific exercises apparently had a positive effect on scoliosis in mature adolescents (Wan et al. 2005).

Recently, two RCTs on conservative treatment have been published, one on corrective exercises (Monticone et al. 2014) and the other on bracing (Weinstein et al. 2013). Therefore, conservative treatment is now supported by evidence on Level I.

In several systematic reviews of the entire treatment spectrum, including surgery, bracing is seen as effective, scoliosis-specific exercise is gaining momentum, and although surgery is the most popular and widely prescribed treatment remedy, recently questions have been raised regarding its necessity based on long-term complications (Weiss and Goodall 2008, Westrick and Ward 2011, Weiss, Moramarco and Moramarco 2013). With this in mind, it is with firm resolve that we commit ourselves to the conservative treatment of scoliosis, especially since no significant side effects or risks have been noted for conservative, active physical rehabilitation techniques specific to scoliotic curve patterns.

Idiopathic scoliosis is classified as infantile, juvenile or adolescent and is determined by the age of initial diagnosis (Winter 1995). The non-idiopathic forms of scoliosis that occur less frequently are, according to Winter (1995):

1. Neuromuscular (neuropathic, myopathic)
2. Congenital
3. Neurofibromatosis
4. Mesenchymal changes (Marfan, Ehlers-Danlos, and others)
5. Osteochondrodystrophy
6. Other rare forms of symptomatic scoliosis (Winter 1995)

Genetic defects (e.g. Prader-Willi syndrome, Fig. 1.6) also play a role (Weiss and Goodall 2009).

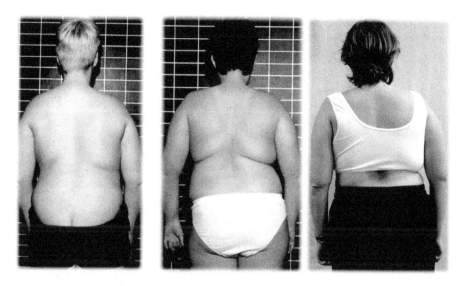

Fig. 1.6: Patients with Prader-Willi syndrome, involving various expressions of a genetic defect. Generally, obesity is present and often an insatiable appetite. Even though the patient tends to be of short stature, patients with Prader-Willi syndrome often have severe scoliosis (Weiss and Goodall 2009).

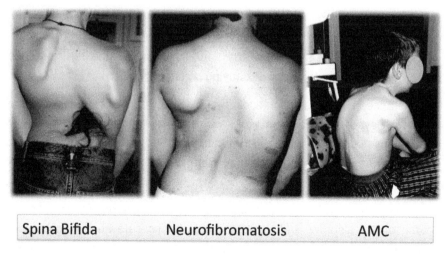

Spina Bifida   Neurofibromatosis   AMC

Fig. 1.7: Various forms of scoliosis. *Left:* ambulatory patient with meningomyelocele without a skin defect, but with considerable hair growth in the area over the defect. *Center:* right convex thoracic scoliosis in a boy with neurofibromatosis. The café au lait spots on the skin are typical. *Right:* boy with arthogryposis multiplex congenital (AMC) with typical kyphoscoliosis.

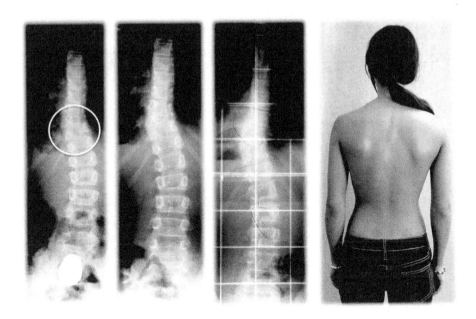

Fig. 1.8: *Left:* x-ray images of development without progression in a girl with congenital scoliosis without any treatment between age 10 and 14. *Right:* the clinical image once growth was complete (Kaspiris et al. 2011).

By definition, idiopathic scoliosis involves curvatures of the spine in otherwise healthy children and adolescents. In contrast, we refer to non-idiopathic scoliosis as symptomatic or even syndromic, since its occurrence can be directly attributed to an underlying disease.

For instance, neuromuscular scoliosis is linked to a disturbance in the nervous system (neuropathic), such as cerebral paresis or meningomyelocele (Fig. 1.7). An example of a subform of myopathic scoliosis is associated with muscular dystrophy or arthrogryposis multiplex congenital (AMC).

Scoliosis with neurofibromatosis is characterized by a rapidly progressive course of the disorder and exhibits characteristic café au lait spots (Fig. 1.7). Because of the potential for rapid progression, the prognosis for symptomatic scoliosis is rather different among the various forms of scoliosis and difficult to predict. Follow-up examinations every three months are advisable during times of growth, as with idiopathic scoliosis. Surgery should not be considered as the first option when there are conservative

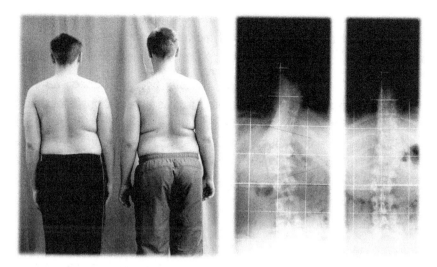

Fig. 1.9: Monozygotic twins with different forms and severity of congenital scoliosis in the x-ray image, but clinically without considerable deformity and therefore not requiring treatment due to having reached physical maturity (Kaspiris et al. 2008).

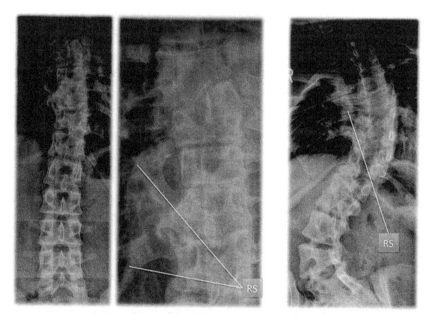

Fig. 1.10: Two patients with congenital scoliosis and rib synostosis (RS). Nearly at the end of bone maturation, the spinal column of the patient on the *left* side is practically straight despite proven rib synostosis. *Center* image is an enlarged view of part of the left image. *Right:* rib synostosis with severe deformity involving multiple segments.

treatment options, particularly since evidence for surgery is lacking (Cheuk et al. 2012) and there are reports of high complication rates (Weiss and Goodall 2008).

With congenital scoliosis, formation defects (wedge-shaped vertebrae, hemivertebrae) need to be differentiated from segmentation defects (one-sided bar formation, rib synostosis). Frequently, formation defects occur hand-in-hand with segmentation defects. Many cases of congenital scoliosis are benign, often requiring no treatment (Fig. 1.8 and Fig. 1.9). Segmentation defects are not necessarily progressive, even if an unfavorable prognosis is assumed when synostosis involves multiple segments (Fig. 1.10).

As far as the clinical appearance is concerned, congenital scoliosis is sometimes inconspicuous (Fig. 1.8 and Fig. 1.9) but can lead to considerable deformities, especially in conjunction with segmentation defects (Fig. 1.11).

The often recommended early operative treatment of congenital scoliosis is usually unnecessary for balanced deformities and not necessarily successful for more severe deformities (Fig. 1.12). The high complication rate after surgery (Weiss and Goodall 2008) and the lack of evidence of long-term post-operative development through the end of adolescence (Kaspiris et al. 2011) makes the case against surgery as a first resort for patients with congenital scoliosis.

Consequently, the primary treatment indication for symptomatic and syndromic scoliosis is the conservative option. A brace is the primary treatment approach during phases of intense growth and specific physical rehabilitation during all phases when growth is expected (Weiss and Goodall 2009, Weiss 2012, Kaspiris et al. 2011).

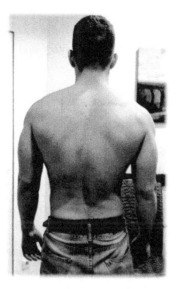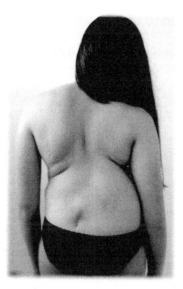

Fig. 1.11: *Left:* a young man with a thoracolumbar formation defect. The thoracolumbar kyphosis in the affected section of the spinal column stands out, while the lateral deviation is not terribly conspicuous. *Right:* adolescent with rib synostosis (see also Fig. 1.10 right) and severe deformity. The first author indicated an operation for this patient. The operation was declined due to considerable neurological risk after an MRT examination was performed by the spinal surgeon.

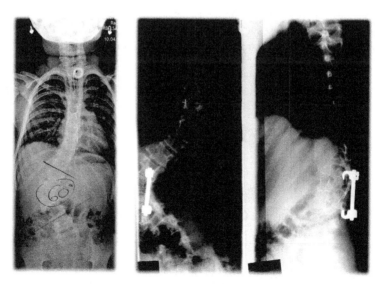

Fig. 1.12: Congenital scoliosis in a small child with a Cobb angle of 60° initially. After surgery he progressed to 85° along with an increase in the lumbar kyphosis.

Reference List

Asher MA, Burton DC. Adolescent idiopathic scoliosis: natural history and long-term treatment effects. Scoliosis. 2006;1(1):2.

Brooks HL, Azen SP, Gerberg EL et al. Scoliosis: a prospective epidemiological study. J Bone Joint Surg [Am]. 1975;57:968.

Caillens JP, Yarrousse Y, Adrey J, Goulesque X. Kreuzschmerz und Lumbalskoliose des Erwachsenen. In: Weiss HR. Wirbelsäulendeformitäten, Bd 1. Heidelberg: Springer; 1991:49–58.

Cheuk DKL, Wong V, Wraige E, Baxter P, Cole A. Surgery for scoliosis in Duchenne muscular dystrophy. Editorial Group: Cochrane Neuromuscular Disease Group. Published Online: 28 Feb 2013. Assessed as up-to-date: 31 Jul 2012.

Cobb JR. Outlines for the study of scoliosis measurements from spinal roentgenograms. Phys Ther. 1948;59:764–765.

Collis DK, Ponseti IV. Long-term followup of patients with idiopathic scoliosis not treated surgically. J Bone Joint Surg [Am]. 1969;51:425–445.

Danielsson AJ, Wiklund I, Pehrsson K, Nachemson AL. Health-related quality of life in patients with adolescent idiopathic scoliosis: a matched followup at least 20 years after treatment with brace or surgery. Euro Spine J. 2001;10:278–288.

Danielsson AJ, Nachemson AL. Radiologic findings and curve progression 11 years after treatment for adolescent idiopathic scoliosis. Comparison of brace and surgical treatment with matching control group of straight individuals. Spine. 2001;26(5):516–552.

DiRocco PJ, Vaccaro P. Cardiopulmonary function in adolescent patients with mild idiopathic scoliosis. Arch Phys Med Rehabil. 1988;69:198–201.

Duriez J. Evolution de la scoliose idiopathique chez l'adulte. Acta Orthop Belg. 1967;33:547–550.

Hawes M, O'Brien J. The transformation of spinal curvature into spinal deformity: pathological processes and implications for treatment. Scoliosis. 2006, Mar 31;1(1):3.

Heine J, Meister R. Quantitative Untersuchungen der Lungenfunktion und der arteriellen Blutgase bei jugendlichen Skoliotikern mit Hilfe eines funktionsdiagnostischen Minimalprograms. Z Orthop. 1972;110:56–62.

Heine J. Die Lumbalskoliose. Stuttgart: Enke; 1980.

Henke G. Rückenverkrümmungen bei Jugendlichen. Bern: Huber; 1982:90–91.

Kaspiris A, Grivas TB, Weiss HR. Congenital scoliosis in monozygotic twins: case report and review of possible factors contributing to its development. Scoliosis. 2008 Nov 18;3:17.

Kaspiris A, Grivas TB, Weiss HR, Turnbull D. Surgical and conservative treatment of patients with congenital scoliosis: a search for long-term results. Scoliosis. 2011 Jun 4;6:12.

Lonstein JE, Carlson JM. The prediction of curve progression in untreated idiopathic scoliosis during growth. J Bone Joint Surg. 1984;66A:1061–1071.

Meister R. Atemfunktion und Lungenkreislauf bei thorakaler Skoliose. Stuttgart: Thieme; 1980: 82–96.

Monticone M, Ambrosini E, Cazzaniga D, Rocca B, Ferrante S. Active self-correction and task-oriented exercises reduce spinal deformity and improve quality of life in subjects with mild adolescent idiopathic scoliosis. Results of a randomised controlled trial. Eur Spine J. 2014 Feb 28. [Epub ahead of print]

Negrini S, Minozzi S, Bettany-Saltikov J, Zaina F, Chockalingam N, Grivas TB, Kotwicki T, Maruyama T, Romano M, Vasiliadis ES: Braces for idiopathic scoliosis in adolescents. Cochrane Database Syst Rev. 2010 Jan 20;(1):CD006850.

Perdriolle R, Vidal J. Thoracic idiopathic scoliosis curve, evolution and prognosis. Spine. 1985;10:785–791.

Pehrsson K, Larsson S, Oden A, et al. Long-term followup of patients with untreated scoliosis. A study of mortality, causes of death, and symptoms. Spine. 1992;17:1091–1096.

Rogala EJ, Drummond DS, Gurr J. Scoliosis: incidence and natural history. A prospective epidemiological study. J Bone Joint Surg. 1978;[Am]60:173–176.

Romano M, Minozzi S, Bettany-Saltikov J, Zaina F, Chockalingam N, Kotwicki T, Maier-Hennes A, Negrini S. Exercises for adolescent idiopathic scoliosis. Cochrane Database Syst Rev. 2012 Aug 15;8:CD007837.

Sahlstrand T, Lidström J. Equilibrium factors as predictors of the prognosis in adolescent idiopathic scoliosis. Clin Orthop. 1980;152: 232.

van Loon PJ, Kühbauch BA, Thunnissen FB: Forced lordosis on the thoracolumbar junction can correct coronal plane deformity in adolescents with double major curve pattern idiopathic scoliosis. Spine. 2008, Apr 1;33(7):797–801.

Wan L, Wang G-X, Bian R. Exercise therapy in treatment of essential S-shaped scoliosis: evaluation of Cobb angle in breast and lumbar segment through a followup of half a year. Chinese J Clin Rehabil. 2005;9:82-84.

Weber B, Smyth JP, Briscoe WA, et al. Pulmonary function in asymptomatic adolescents with idiopathic scoliosis. Am Rev Respir Dis. 1975;111:389–397.

Weinstein SL. Adolescent idiopathic scoliosis: prevalence, natural history, treatment indications. Iowa: University of Iowa Printing Service; 1985.

Weinstein SL. Idiopathic scoliosis. Natural history. Spine. 1986;11:780.

Weinstein SL, Dolan LA, Wright JG, Dobbs MB. Effects of bracing in adolescents with idiopathic scoliosis. N Engl J Med. 2013 Oct 17;369(16):1512-21. doi: 10.1056/NEJMoa1307337.

Weiss HR. Scoliosis-related pain in adults – treatment influences. Eur J Phys Rehabil Med. 1993;3:91–94.

Weiss HR, Verres C, Steffan K, Heckel I. Scoliosis and pain – is there any relationship? In: Research into Spinal Deformities II Edited by: I.A.F. Stokes. 293 - 296 IOS Press, Amsterdam, 1999.

Weiss HR, Klein R. Improving excellence in scoliosis rehabilitation: a controlled study of matched pairs. Pediatr Rehabil. 2006;9:3. 190–200 Jul/Sep.

Weiss HR, Goodall D. Rate of complications in scoliosis surgery – a systematic review of the Pub Med literature. Scoliosis. 2008;3:08.

Weiss HR, Goodall D. Scoliosis in patients with Prader Willi Syndrome – comparisons of conservative and surgical treatment. Scoliosis. 2009 May 6;4:10.

Weiss HR. Brace treatment in infantile/juvenile patients with progressive scoliosis is worthwhile. Stud Health Technol Inform. 2012;176:383-6.

Weiss HR, Moramarco M. Scoliosis – treatment indications according to current evidence. OA Musculoskeletal Medicine. 2013 Mar 01;1(1):1.

Weiss HR, Moramarco M, Moramarco K. Risks and long-term complications of adolescent idiopathic scoliosis surgery vs. non-surgical and natural history outcomes. Hard Tissue. 2013 Apr 30;2(3):27.

Weiss HR, Seibel S. Region of interest in the radiological follow-up of patients with scoliosis Hard Tissue. 2013 Jun 01;2(4):33.

Westrick ER, Ward WT. Adolescent idiopathic scoliosis: 5-year to 20-year evidence-based surgical results. J Pediatr Orthop. 2011 Jan-Feb;31(1 Suppl):S61-8.

Winter RB. Classification and terminology In: Lonstein J, Bradford D, Winter R, Ogilvie J, editors. Moe's textbook of scoliosis and other spinal deformities. Philadelphia: WB Saunders 1995 p39-44.

2 History

Scoliosis was recognized as early as the 5th century BC when Hippocrates (460-375 BC) described scoliosis and its treatment (Fig. 2.1). His belief was that one of the causes of the deformation of the vertebrae was the luxation of the spine. He tried to counteract this luxation using mechanical devices. In the process, he made use of the Hippocratic luxation table (Vasiliades et al. 2009). The Romans also recognized the Hippocratic luxation table. Galenos (130-201 AD) described spinal deformations in the following way: kyphosis (curvature to the rear), lordosis (curvature to the front), and scoliosis (lateral curvature).

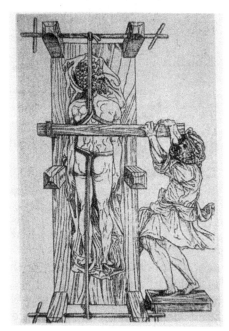

Fig. 2.1: The "luxation table" from Hippocrates (see also Vasiliades et al. 2009).

In the 16th century, the Hippocratic luxation table was still recognized as an effective method. In the same century, however, the first supportive braces were described and would go on to be promoted by Paré (Paré 1840). It was only at the beginning of the 19th century and particularly at the beginning of the 20th century when a systematic orthopedic physiotherapeutic method was introduced. This physio-therapeutic treatment was supported by the founding of various orthopedic institutions. These institutions which made time-intensive treatment possible were a prerequisite for successful education concerning posture. In these special institutions, brace fitting occurred under the supervision of a doctor, often for hours on end. In addition, gymnastic exercises were carried out, frequently with the help of mechanical correction devices that were specially constructed for the treatment of scoliosis (Fig. 2.2-2.3). Residency in these establishments was very expensive and few people could afford such treatment.

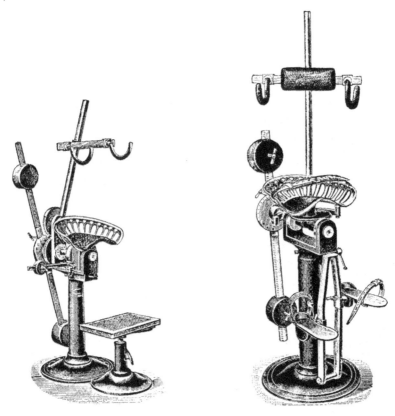

Fig. 2.2: Representation of two correction (redressment) devices for spinal gymnastics. The trunk moved against the seat area, which was why these devices were described by Schanz (1904) as "trunk pendulums."

In the 19th century, Zander (1893) tried to overcome the problem of large staff costs with the construction of diverse equipment. Instead of manual resistance from the therapist, he employed suitable devices with resistance for the patient to overcome which could be increased or decreased as one desired, with the extent of the resistance being set using weights.

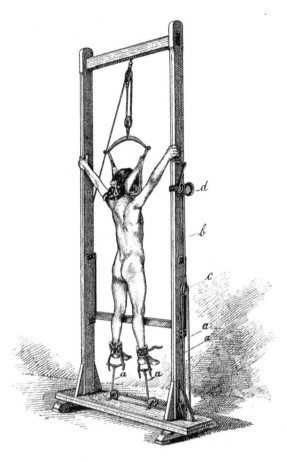

Fig. 2.3: Correction devices for suspension and correction in preparation for the plaster bandage treatment (Schanz, 1904).

Lorenz (1886) and Hoffa (1905) developed treatment in the passive upright position. In this treatment, one attempts to achieve a correction of the spine by way of passive reshaping. Lorenz introduced reshaping exercises, which were executed with the assistance of specialized equipment (Fig. 2.4). Hoffa (1905) introduced active exercises in the upright position for the treatment of scoliosis. Parallel to the manual upright attempts, therapy was also developed which utilized machines, as used by Wullstein (1902). Patients were initially stretched using various instruments, and, in order to stabilize the spine, patients were immobilized in plaster or wore braces for many years. Klapp developed his own method before 1905. This method was expanded into a physiotherapeutic system by the development of specific exercises that were tailored to the various forms of scoliosis. He raised awareness that muscles, bones, and ligaments can only be strengthened through functional use. Thus, his system was a forerunner of functional physiotherapy. The Klapp technique consisted of actively mobilizing the spine and simultaneously strengthening the musculature to help retain flexibility. Klapp observed that good results could only be achieved if these exercises were carried out for at least two hours a day. His method had many enthusiastic supporters, but soon had its critics too, some of whom pointed to possible deterioration of the countercurve due to his method (Lange 1913), while others generally criticized the mobilization of the spine (Haglund 1916).

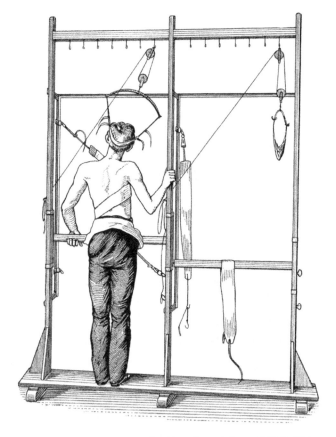

Fig. 2.4: Modification of the Lorenz spiral cables, from Schanz (1904). This was a passive correction device used several times a day to achieve a corrective effect for treatment taking place over the course of many months.

In Schanz's book (1904) concerning the load-bearing deformities of the spine, he provides a good overview of the possible treatments that were available at the time. He doesn't neglect questions concerning everyday activities, and, in particular, he provides information concerning the furniture in schools. He also presents the benefits of massage and remedial gymnastics (Fig. 2.5), which, in his opinion, can be summarized as follows: massage and remedial gymnastics can contribute to the minimizing of the static demands on the spine. They do this by reducing the period of time in which the spine is in a position of fatigue and therefore subject to relatively high static demands. Massage and gymnastics can also contribute to an increase of the static performance of the spine. By improving the general condition of the body and strengthening the spinal musculature, they help to bring about an increase in the rigidity of the osseous tissue in the spine.

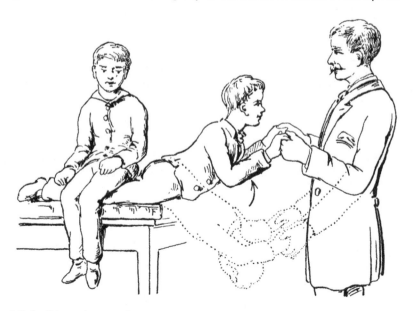

Fig. 2.5: Staff-intensive upright exercises to strengthen the trunk muscles (Schanz 1904).

Schanz valued the advantages of massage and remedial gymnastics all the more since there were apparently no significant disadvantages to the techniques.

Brace treatment was introduced, as well as redressment (correction) devices that were intended to support the "plaster bandage treatment." After correction therapy in the plaster mold, very good results were achieved.

Interestingly, the brace treatment available at that time differs from contemporary treatment only slightly. The "portative correction device" also shares similarities to the dynamic correction brace (DCB) used today.

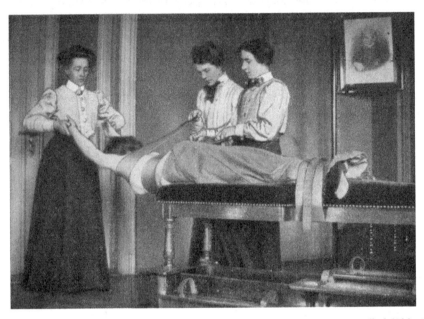

Fig. 2.6: Staff-intensive physiotherapy for spinal deformities – the strap is pulled (Oldevig 1913).

Swedish remedial gymnastics according to Ling's method (1924) grew in popularity at the beginning of the 20th century. Ling used resistance exercises in sitting, standing, and hanging positions, as well as lying on the front and the back. Oldevig (1913), who was instrumental in the introduction of Swedish remedial gymnastics in Germany, had recognized the disadvantage of these resistance exercises which always needed to be carried out under the guidance of at least one doctor or physiotherapist (Fig. 2.5-2.6).

With his belt exercises (Fig. 2.7-2.8), Oldevig tried to isolate individual curvatures and work on them in that way. The aim of the belt exercises was to trigger muscle activity. Oldevig believed that muscle activity could be achieved more conveniently, more precisely, and more effectively through belt exercises than through any other method. He saw the "gymnast" as a modeler who reshapes the living body. He therefore demanded from this gymnast a high level of independent reflection, much feeling, and visual judgment. The exercises he developed are based on anatomical principles and it was of absolute importance to him that compensatory curvatures not be increased during the exercises.

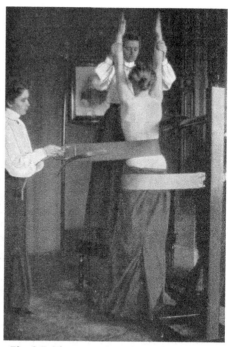

Fig. 2.7: Therapy involving pulling a strap in a standing position, with extra staff assisting (Oldevig 1913).

For Lange (1907), scoliosis was a disruption of the muscular balance. He constructed various resistance devices with which he wanted to achieve an overcorrection of the spine. The patient had to rebend the spine on the concave side against the resistance of the device in order to achieve the desired overcorrection.

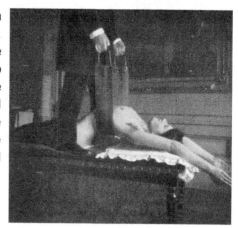

Fig. 2.8: Lordosis exercises for kyphosis according to the Oldevig method (Oldevig 1913).

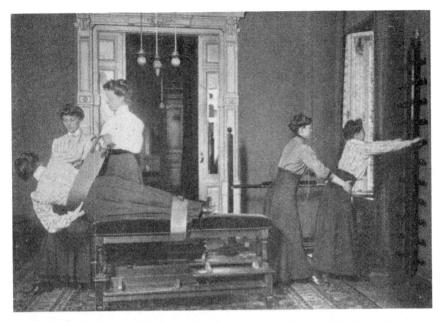

Fig. 2.9: Typical setting of the correction exercises, according to Oldevig, at the wooden bars and on the exercise bench (Oldevig 1913).

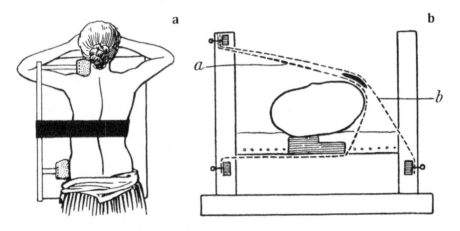

Fig. 2.10: (a) A schematic representation of the three-point principle for correction in a belt device and **(b)** schematic representation of correction straps that looped the costal hump dorsolaterally (Lange 1907).

Everyday activities played an important role. Lange visualized the scoliosis curvature using his "diopter" and could thus monitor the success of the treatment. The goal of his treatment was to correct the insufficiency in the erector spinae muscles. He was of the opinion that there were two conditions that had to be satisfied in order to tackle scoliosis effectively:

1. The scoliosis-affected spine needed to be re-bent forcefully, both actively and passively (Fig. 2.9, 2.10);

2. The devices used for the active and passive overcorrection needed to be as simple as possible (Fig. 2.11).

Lange also observed the countercurve and stated that an overcorrection must be strictly limited to the section of the spine that was distorted. It was for this reason that he was not able to sympathize with "the original idea of the highly esteemed Bonn-based surgeon Klapp," who wanted to heal scoliosis using crawling.

Blencke (1913) was an advocate of the more specific treatment approach for scoliosis. He distinguished between remedial gymnastics for general treatment and a form of correction gymnastics for a direct influence on the pathological form of spinal deformities (Fig. 2.12-2.13). He rejected the idea that just anyone or even just any gymnastics teacher could provide treatment for scoliosis. For serious cases of scoliosis, he believed that

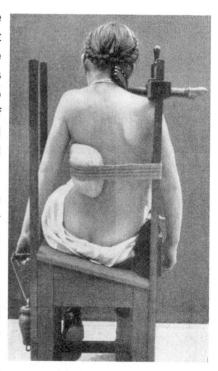

Fig. 2.11 A patient sitting in a three-point correction device (Lange 1907).

asymmetric exercises were indispensable (Fig. 2.14a, b). Just as Schultheß did, he viewed special orthopedic gymnastics for the treatment of scoliosis as work to be tailored to the individual case. Treatment involved an overcoming of resistances in specially chosen positions, with certain parts of

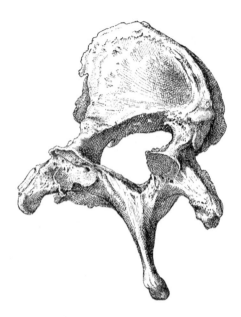

Fig. 2.12: The torsion pattern of a thoracic vertebra with scoliosis. The vertebral body tends to the right whilst the zygapophyseal joint lies more to the left and the spinous process points to the right. Furthermore, there is a wedge-shaped formation that is not shown on this image (Blencke 1913).

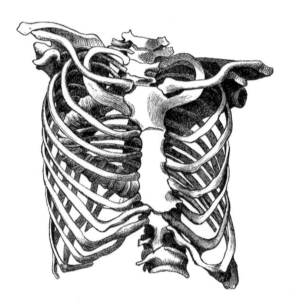

Fig. 2.13: Torsion of the ribcage with thoracic scoliosis. (Blencke 1913).

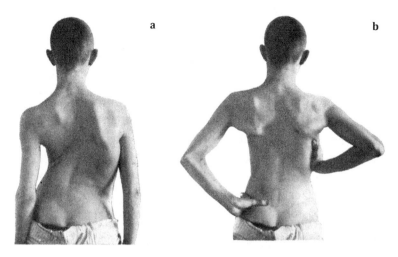

Fig. 2.14: (a) A patient with right thoracic scoliosis and left lumbar counterswing before the exercise. **(b)** The patient in the auto-correction, which was to be carried out several times a day (Blencke 1913).

the skeleton being held in a fixed position with the elimination of certain secondary movements and undesired side effects. Blencke (1913) also viewed the Klapp crawling exercises in a negative light, since, in his opinion, gymnastic scoliosis treatment needed to be tailored to the individual.

Around the end of the second decade of the 20th century, Katharina Schroth developed her three-dimensional scoliosis treatment. Her own body had been deformed by scoliosis and it was by looking at the way that it reacted that she developed specific corrective mechanisms and a corrective breathing technique that she named "rotational breathing" (Fig. 2.15a-b). Along with the rotational breathing technique, Schroth's holistic principle was new to the treatment of scoliosis. Katharina Schroth wanted to influence scoliosis via a change in the entire feeling of the body.

With the opening of the first institute in Meißen in 1921, Schroth's three-dimensional treatment for scoliosis enjoyed increased popularity. For the first time scoliosis wasn't simply seen in a mechanical light – although the mechanics by no means played an inferior role. Katharina Schroth introduced for the first time sensorimotor kinesthetic principles to the treatment options of scoliosis. These principles use the most active erection possible to provide a sense of awareness in order to avoid curvature-inducing behavior in one's daily routine (Fig. 2.16 and 2.17). Breathing was also integrated as a crucial factor in the correction of scoliosis not only of the ribcage, but also of the lumbar spinal region (Schroth 1924, 1929, 1931, 1935). After introducing these principles, treatment lasting three to six months would be carried out with the most serious cases of scoliosis.

The successful treatment of curvatures, some of which were very significant and rigid, can be seen in the first publications from the institute that Katharina Schroth founded (Fig. 2.15 - 2.17). However, in a report whose contents only became known after the Second World War, Prof. Schede from Leipzig criticized the treatment as early as the 20s, describing the treatment as "charlatanism that people must be warned against."

This criticism was so influential that it led to the removal of Franz Schroth – Katharina's husband – from his official post position. His wife's work was supposedly scandalous and unworthy of an official. However, there were also many positive voices from the medical profession that ultimately led to Franz's reinstatement after a disciplinary inquiry.

In 1924, Katharina Schroth published the small volume *Die Atmungskur.* The Essen-based Dr. Grewers wrote the following in the foreword:

> "Personally, I can already judge that which I have seen and I will never fail to recommend this technique to patients in certain cases, since I know that it will be of help to them where everything else has failed them. I do not believe I am saying too much when I claim that this remedial system has a full medical grounding and that a medical practitioner free of prejudice can use it side-by-side with the existing remedial system."

The volume was not intended necessarily for those suffering from scoliosis, but rather contains information for exercises for all patients suffering from collapsed posture. However, Katharina Schroth makes it clear that she addresses the treatment of scoliosis with particular focus. This is clear in the following description of treatment:

> "I then brought out the left side slowly but surely using one-sided breathing and many types of gymnastic exercises. Since there was a double curvature, I of course had to be careful that none of the exercises helped one part but damaged the other. It is often the case that canceling-out exercises must be carried out. Meticulous observation and many years of experience also allow one to avoid these pitfalls."

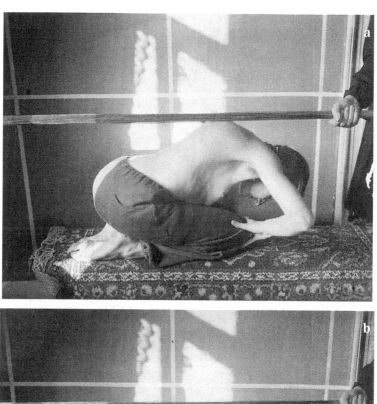

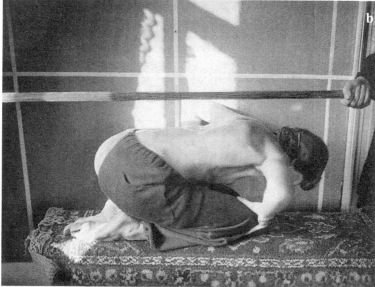

Fig. 2.15: Execution of the rotational breathing technique with a severe thoracic distortion (**a**) before the exercise and (**b**) during the exercise. Positive results were observed after many months of treatment.

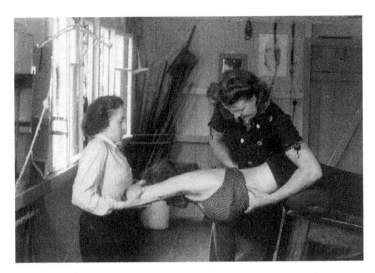

Fig. 2.16: Strengthening the feeling of posture via the use of so-called "redressment (corrective) grasps" and "breath grasps" to improve the corrective movement during exercising.

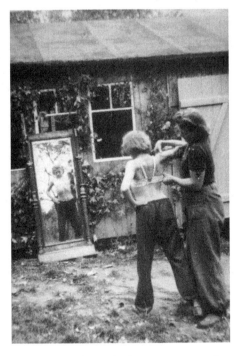

Fig. 2.17: Use of mirror control in order to facilitate auto-correction with the assistance of breathing.

In 1929, Katharina Schroth presented her increasingly holistic approach in a second illustrated brochure:

"Why is it so often the case that gymnastic efforts to straighten out the spine of a child suffering in this way so often result in failure? Because one approaches the child in a far too mechanical way, far too exercise-oriented, without first investigating the difficulties the child experiences in life, the unendurable problems they have – problems that might well seem insignificant to an adult. Getting the external person to stand up straight and erect their spine will only be possible if you first allow the inner person to 'stand up straight,' to give them hope, to allow them to 'breathe out.' Here, language shows itself to be much smarter than the current materialistically minded generation of, let us say, practitioners who view the human as a machine."

In *Naturmedizin* (Natural Doctor), a publication from 1931, Katharina Schroth wrote the following about the rotational breathing technique:

"It is challenged on many sides that one can control one's breathing so precisely that it will go where we want it to go. To achieve it, the teacher must help the pupil to develop a sense of control for the right load and the wrong load, for the proper orientation of the rib joints at the right location."

The principle of "helping the patient to help themselves" is also present in the same article:

"If one considers how terrible the lot of those who suffer from spinal deformations is, how ostracized they must feel simply due to their appearance, how limited they are in their professional life, how reduced their joy in life is, then one must accept that in order to achieve an improvement to this situation – something that is perfectly possible – a brief education with expert instruction must first create a foundation that can then be built upon at home in self-treatment."

On the subject of "body feeling," we find the following statement from Katharina Schroth in a special edition of a journal from the upper Ore Mountains region in 1935:

"It is self-evident that the patient must be activated in each and every sense: bodily, mentally, and emotionally; that they themselves must take on the struggle against their suffering – for the character, this educational influence brings with it intense repercussions. With precise and specific work one can unlock the potential to develop the patient's body feeling and to generate a sense of the body on a higher level, so that even work involving layers of muscle buried deep under other layers is under command and can be carried out precisely. This is a scenario whose possibility of fulfillment leaves even highly educated professional gymnasts lost for words."

There is very little written information about the treatment system developed by Gocht and Gessner. Gocht (1909) had concerned himself initially with the equipment-based treatment of scoliosis; however, the exercises based on Gocht and Gessner's work were developed after 1925 at the Charité Hospital in Berlin. Mater (1957) wrote the following on the subject:

"The scoliosis exercises that Gocht and Debrunner described in their book *Orthopedic Therapy* from 1925 are not the same as those that are carried out today. In this book, above all it is corrections of the spine that are described with the patient in a passive role. Treatment is through hand pressure against the costal hump and thus a movement of the trunk against the pelvis, or in the case of lumbar scoliosis, a pelvic inclination on the concave side via re-location and relief of the affected leg. Gocht describes these as an active static recurving. The exercises that Ms. Gessner arranged at the Berlin Charité Hospital in later years, which are in principle still broadly in use today, are actually exercises taken from Swedish remedial gymnastics. Here, one tries to counter the lateral inclination and twisting of the spine simply through active muscle work in the form of stretches and the isolated tensing of the convex side transverse musculature."

For Hug (1921), the degenerated muscle fibers have a central role in scoliosis. We find him saying, for example, "the earlier the onset of scoliosis, the more drastic the bodily deformation." His principle for treatment is the "temporary overcorrection on the other side." At least from a mechanical perspective, he is in agreement with Lange and Schroth here.

For Port (1922), the musculature is also of key importance. He was of the opinion that the development of rachitic scoliosis was dependent upon the condition of the musculature. For him, this meant that the practitioner's entire attention must be turned towards the musculature and that measures of redressment and supportive braces only be worn for the sake of the musculature.

Farkas (1925) noted that with thoracic scoliosis a lordosis can be observed. On the other hand, he noted that kyphosis had the opposite effect. He describes the paradoxical phenomenon that, in actual fact, the costal hump is increased by lordosis, reduced through kyphosis and therefore, in terms of the apparent degree of costal hump, lordosis and kyphosis behave inversely. He was of the opinion that the development of "habitual" scoliosis took place in the same way and was caused and promoted by the same factors as physiological scoliosis, namely from the mechanics of walking. There is a quotation from him that the admonishers amongst those involved in therapy should bear in mind:

> "A child that continues to sit improperly, despite "reminders," does not get scoliosis, but rather already suffers from it. The reclining position of a child suffering from scoliosis is indeed a scoliotic position, because it demands the least possible work and because all other reclining positions are associated with effort by the child and are therefore no longer actual comfortable reclining positions."

This opinion is just as relevant today as it was then and should also be taken into consideration in the conceptual development of treatment for scoliosis.

On the subject of therapeutic setting of goals, Farkas said the following: "The principle of functional therapy for scoliosis is based on the restriction of damaged functions." Farkas believed that the contraction of the spine could be corrected, in terms of inclination. He went on to explain that one could only influence the portion of the costal hump that arose from the rotation of the trunk.

Heuer (1927) summarizes the work concerning the etiology of scoliosis and develops a self-sufficient model of scoliosis.

Despite Katharina Schroth's scoliosis treatment being received warmly in many circles, Lempert and Brodermann (1931) still favored the Klapp exercises. However, the authors were not critical of the exercises and expressed no position with respect to the possible deterioration of countercurves as a result of this treatment method – the reason this method came under fire from critics two decades earlier.

At the beginning of the 20th century, Egon von Niederhöffer also concerned himself with the biomechanics of the back musculature in cases of scoliosis. In her publications from 1929 and 1936, Luise von Niederhöffer does not yet exhibit a physiotherapeutic concept. It was only in 1942 that the Niederhöffer treatment principle was presented along with a sequence of exercises (Fig. 2.18) – this would later be refined by Becker.

After the Second World War, Katharina Schroth and her daughter Christa relocated to the west and founded a new institute in what was then known as Sobernheim, following the wards in Bad Steben and Bad Kreuznach. This institute was initially exclusively private, but was then run as a sanatorium from the beginning of the 70s. Here, Katharina Schroth's three-dimensional scoliosis treatment was developed further and quickly became more and more well known. Before the end of the 70s, the effect of stationary intensive rehabilitation of the breathing function was studied with a comparison group. Götze (1976) was able to show that this kind of intensive program not only increased cardio-

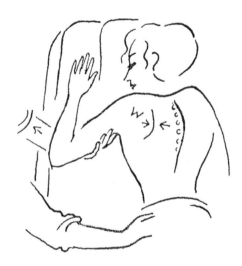

Fig. 2.18: Description of von Niederhöffer's treatment principle. Above the surface musculature a correction movement was carried out on the spine with the help of the thoracic concave side arm. This is contrary to the three-dimensional scoliosis treatment developed by Schroth where the ribcage is first corrected and the thoracic convex side arm is pulled against the ribcage correction over to the thoracic convex side, in order to correct the cranial section (modified from Weber and Hirsch 1986).

pulmonary performance, but also the vital capacity; the vital capacity showed no significant change after a four-week aerobic fitness program.

Despite being led by medical professionals, the establishment – which had been named the Katharina Schroth Clinic in the 80s – became the target of multiple accusations from critics of the method. Using a supposedly academically led "method fight," they tried to annul this concept, which was becoming more and more successful. After this conflict had been overcome, the method received general recognition from everyone in the orthopedic world and from German insurance companies.

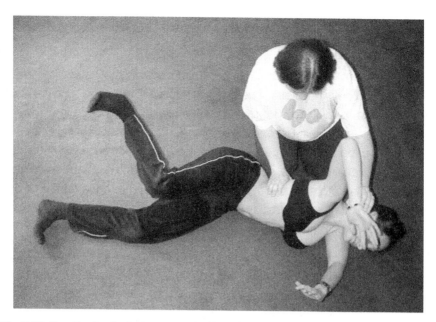

Fig. 2.19: Exercise for the facilitation of reflex turning, developed by Vojta.

In the 50s, Vaclav Vojta began developing a treatment for children with cerebal palsy based on kinesiologic methods. In the 60s and 70s (Vojta, 1965), his treatment began gaining the interest of German therapists. By the end of the 70s, Vojta's treatment was widespread and scoliosis was also being treated using his approach. With this method, the belief was that, with the assistance of facilitation of the reflex movements, the muscular imbalance that exists in patients suffering from scoliosis can be compensated through central mechanisms. Many mistakenly believed that the correction could be predominantly traced back to the increase in activity of the segmental dorsal musculature, which is partially degenerated in the case of scoliosis (Fig. 2.19).

At the beginning of the 80s, Hanke introduced the E-technique (E-Technik), based upon Vojta's principles. In a horizontal position, he tried to straighten out the costal hump via tension exercises and, at the same time, stabilize the posture, which had been altered by the central reactions.

Today, apart from Katharina Schroth's three-dimensional scoliosis treatment, the old treatments no longer play a significant role in Germany because they have not been continually developed over time. This is also the case with Scharll's scoliosis treatment, which experienced a renaissance in the 80s (Weber and Hirsch 1986).

In the outpatient setting, Schroth's three-dimensional scoliosis treatment is spreading. The physiotherapeutic treatment methods based on developmental kinesiology (Vojta and Hanke) are still employed in Germany to some degree as well. Beyond these, numerous approaches were used in the past to expand the range of treatment methods for scoliosis (Ozarcuk 1994), but over time these have been abandoned due to imprecision and inefficiency. Therefore, in the outpatient field, we can in good faith limit our selection of suitable physical rehabilitation methods to those introduced above and the subsequent developments they experienced.

Undoubtably, in other countries and other continents there are and have been effective developments for the conservative treatment of scoliosis, perhaps many hundreds or thousands of years old.

However, perhaps the readers will forgive the first author for limiting his sketches to the developments within the German-speaking world. At the time of publication, no comprehensive international multilingual sources were available.

Recently, several developments on the international level have been marketed aggressively, such as yoga, SEAS, or Dobomed (Fusco et al. 2011), although these approaches apparently make do without using a systematic system of correction. If, however, we bear in mind that with brace provision we are absolutely concerned with the correction effect (Landauer et al. 2003), then we should focus on methods that are inherently corrective, such as Side-Shift, Schroth, and the Schroth Best Practice program® (Borysov and Borysov 2012, Pugacheva 2012, Monticone et al. 2014, Lee 2014) when choosing which rehabilitative method to pursue.

In all probability, the future will be governed by treatment approaches that are simpler and easier, but without compromising effectiveness. New pedagogical approaches must take into account that today's adolescent patient is unlike the youth of times past who regularly underwent six-week stationary intensive rehabilitation. Experiential learning should be incorporated and treatment approaches which align methodology to the constantly changing traits of the patients are essential for a positive outcome.

It is safe to assume that Katharina Schroth's three-dimensional scoliosis treatment and its subsequent development, the Schroth Best Practice program®, are the most widely used forms of treatment across the globe. Books on the subject have already been translated into many languages. The upcoming sub-chapter will focus on the history of Katharina Schroth's three-dimensional scoliosis treatment drawn in part from a publication from Weiss, 2011.

Reference List

Blencke A. Orthopädische Sonderturnkurse. Stuttgart, Enke; 1913.

Borysov M, Borysov A. Scoliosis short-term rehabilitation (SSTR) according to 'Best Practice' standards – are the results repeatable? Scoliosis. 2012 Jan 17;7(1):1.

Farkas A. Über die Bedingungen und auslösenden Momente bei der Skolioseentwicklung. Stuttgart, Enke; 1925.

Fusco C, Zaina F, Atanasio S, Romano M, Negrini A, Negrini S. Physical exercises in the treatment of adolescent idiopathic scoliosis: an updated systematic review. Physiother Theory Pract 2011; 27(1):80–114.

Gocht. Ein einfacher Extensions und Lordierungsapparat für Rückgratsverkrümmungen. Verhandlung der deutschen Gesellschaft für orthopädische Chirurgie, 8. Kongress. Z. Orthop. 1909;24:289–295.

Götze HG. Die Rehabilitation jugendlicher Skoliose-Patienten. Untersuchungen zur cardiopulmonalen Leistungsfähigkeit und zum Enfluß von Krankengymnastik und Sport (Habilitation Thesis). Westfälische Wilhelms-Universität, Münster. 1976:206–209.

Haglund P. Die Entstehung und Behandlung von Skoliosen. S. Karger Berlin; 1916.

Hanke P. Skoliosebehandlung auf entwicklungskinesiologischer Grundlage in Anlehnung an die Vojta-Therapie. Vortrag am 2.2.1983 in Würzburg. Diskussionsreihe „Krankengymnastische Skoliosetherapie" der Arbeitsgemeinschaft Atemtherapie im ZVK; 1983.

Heuer F. Zur Theorie der Skoliose. Darmstadt, Eduard Roether GmbH; 1927.

Hoffa A. Lehrbuch der orthop. Chirurgie. Berlin; 1905.

Hug O. Thorakoplastik und Skoliose. Stuttgart: Enke; 1921.

Klapp R. Funktionelle Behandlung der Skoliose. Jena: Fischer; 1907.

Landauer F, Wimmer C, Behensky H. Estimating the final outcome of brace treatment for idiopathic thoracic scoliosis at 6-month followup. Pediatr Rehabil. 2003;6(3–4):201–7.

Lange F. Die Behandlung der habituellen Skoliose durch aktive und passive Überkorrektur. Stuttgart, Enke; 1907.

Lange F et al. Die Skoliose. Ergebn. Chir. 1913;7:748.

Lee SG. Improvement of curvature and deformity in a sample of patients with Idiopathic Scoliosis with specific exercises. OA Musculoskeletal Medicine. 2014; Mar 12;2(1):6.

Lempert G, Brodermann W. Entstehung und Beseitigung körperlicher Formfehler. Hamburg, Carl A. Langer; 1931.

Ling PH. Zitiert aus Törngren LM: Lehrbuch der Schwedischen Gymnastik. 4. Aufl., Esslingen; 1924.

Lorenz A. Pathologie und Therapie der seitlichen Rückgratverkrümmungen (Scoliosis). Wien: Hölder; 1886.

Mater M. Methoden der heutigen krankengymnastischen Behandlung bei Fehlhaltung und Fehlformen der Wirbelsäule. Z. Krankengymnastik. 1957;9:6–8.

Monticone M, Ambrosini E, Cazzaniga D, Rocca B, Ferrante S. Active self-correction and task-oriented exercises reduce spinal deformity and improve quality of life in subjects with mild adolescent idiopathic scoliosis. Results of a randomised controlled trial. Eur Spine J. 2014 Feb 28. [Epub ahead of print]

Oldevig J. Ein neues Gerät und neue Übungen der Schwedischen Heilgymnastik zur Behandlung von Rückgrats-Verkrümmungen. Berlin, Springer; 1913.

Ozarcuk L. Grundlagen der Skoliosebehandlung mit der propriozeptiven neuromuskulären Fazilitation (PNF). In: Weiss HR (Hrsg) Wirbelsäulendeformitäten Bd. 3, 1994:11–30.

Paré A. Oeuvres complètes. Ed. Par Malgaigné, Tome II, Chap. VIII, 1840:611.

Port K. Über das Wesen der Skoliose. Eine klinische und röntgenologische Studie. Stuttgart: Enke, 1922.

Pugacheva N. Corrective exercises in multimodality therapy of idiopathic scoliosis in children - analysis of six weeks efficiency - pilot study. Stud Health Technol Inform. 2012; 176:365-371.

Schanz A. Die statistischen Belastungsdeformitäten der Wirbelsäule mit besonderer Berücksichtigung der kindlichen Wirbelsäule. Stuttgart: Enke; 1904.

Schroth K. Die Atmungskur. Chemnitz: G. Zimmermann; 1. Auflage; 1924.

Schroth K. Gefahren bei der Behandlung seitlicher Rückgratverkrümmungen. 2. Bild prospekt. Zimmermann, Chemnitz, 1. Auflage; 1929.

Schroth K. Behandlung der Skoliose (Rückgratverkrümmung) durch Atmungsorthopädie. In: Der Naturarzt (Hersg.: Deutscher Bund der Vereine für naturgemäße Lebensund Heilweise Naturheilkunde). 1931: 11–15.

Schroth K. Wie helfen wir den Rückgratverkrümmten? Sonderdruck aus Nr. 143 vom 25. Juni 1935 der „Obererzgebirgischen Zeitung" Buchholz.

Vasiliadis ES, Grivas TB, Kaspiris A. Historical overview of spinal deformities in ancient Greece. Scoliosis. 2009 Feb 25;4:6.

Vojta V. Rehabilitation des spastischen infantilen Syndroms. Eigene Methodik. Beitr Orthop Traumat. 1965;12:557.

von Niederhöffer E. Neue Beobachtungen über die Mechanik der breiten Rückenmuskeln und über deren Beziehungen zur Skoliose. München/Berlin: Verlag Rudolph Müller und Steinicke; 1929.

von Niederhöffer L. Zur Behandlung von Rückgratverkrümmungen. Zeitschrift für Krüppelfürsorge. 1936;29:134.

von Niederhöffer L. Die Behandlung von Rückgratverkrümmungen (Skoliose) nach dem System Niederhöffer. Berlin: Osterwieck; 1942.

Weber M, Hirsch S. Krankengymnastik bei idiopathischer Skoliose. Stuttgart: Fischer; 1986.

Weiss HR. The method of Katharina Schroth – history, principles and current development. Scoliosis. 2011 Aug 30;6:17. doi: 10.1186/1748-7161-6-17.

Wullstein L. Die Skoliose in ihrer Behandlung und Entstehung nach klinischen und experimentellen Studien. Z Orthop. 1902;10:177.

Zander G. Über die Behandlung der habituellen Skoliose mittels mechanischer Gymnastik. Z für Orthop Chir Bd.2; 189:338.

2.1 Katharina Schroth's scoliosis treatment method

Katharina Schroth was born February 22, 1894, in Dresden, Germany. She suffered from moderate scoliosis and underwent treatment with a steel brace at the age of sixteen before she decided to develop a more functional treatment approach.

Inspired by a balloon, she tried to breathe away the deformities of her own trunk by inflating the concavities of her body selectively in front of a mirror. She also tried to "mirror" the deformity by overcorrecting with the help of certain pattern specific corrective movements. She recognized that postural control can only be achieved by changing postural perception.

This new treatment concept consisting of specific postural correction, correction of breathing patterns, and correction of postural perception was introduced at a small institute she had established in Meissen, Germany, with rehabilitation taking place over the course of three months. Beginning in the late 30s and early 40s, she was assisted by her daughter, Christa Schroth, a collaboration that spanned decades.

It wasn't until the late 1980s that the first studies of Schroth methodology were carried out. The patient series for the first prospective controlled trial was derived from the patient samples of 1989–1991.

Over time, the content has evolved and rehabilitation times have changed. Bracing has been introduced and refined for Schroth compatibility to offer patients improved treatment outcomes.

In the last few years, the first author modified the older techniques thereby modernizing the program and reducing training times by adding new forms of postural education such as sagittal correction, activities of daily living (ADL) correction and experiential learning.

While the program is still based on the original approaches of the three-dimensional treatment according to Katharina Schroth – specific postural correction, correction of breathing patterns, and correction of postural perception – the patient is now instructed in a way where these concepts can more easily be applied during daily routines.

The Schroth Method and its evolution

The history of conservative treatment of scoliosis is rather long and leads us back to the original methods of Hippocrates, 460–370 BC (Vasiliades et al. 2009). Although more than 2000 years have passed since the days of Hippocrates, the main approach of conservative scoliosis treatment in the early 20th century was still based on mechanical viewpoints or concepts related to approaches still used today. Correction exercises were used widely throughout Europe during the last two centuries. Some of them requiring three therapists for one patient (Fig. 2.6) during scoliosis correction (Oldevig 1913).

The history of the Schroth method involves the professional work of three generations. The initiation of the program was the result of Katharina Schroth's self study, in part as a result of analyzing her own body, her own spinal function, and the corrective movement patterns. Mirror monitoring took on an important role in the original Schroth program, as it does in current protocols, and allows the patient to synchronize the corrective movement and postural perception with visual feedback (Fig. 2.18). Since breathing and its functional correction play such a key role, her first writings focused on breathing in general (Schroth 1924). Later, she also described the importance of postural perception by the patient and its improvement via specific correction exercises (Schroth 1931, 1935).

The Schroth family history as it relates to scoliosis all began in East Germany early in the last century. Katharina Schroth began her professional life as a teacher at a business and language school. However, she decided to change careers to undergo training at a gymnastics school (predecessors to what we know as a physical therapy education). She immediately recognized that the techniques learned were not specific to scoliosis, however, this allowed her to begin to treat patients like herself.

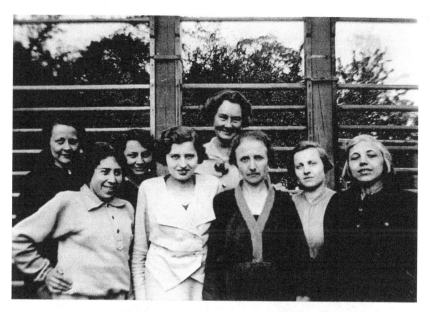

Fig. 2.21: Katharina Schroth (center in the background) seen with her patients in the 30s. [Historical picture from the picture database of Christa Lehnert-Schroth].

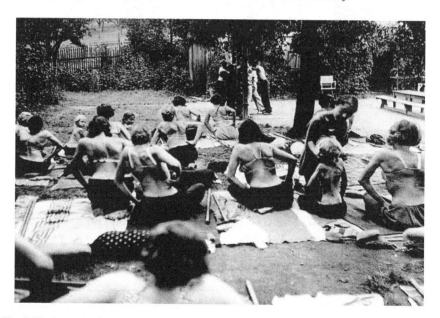

Fig. 2.22: A group of patients with large curvatures exercising in the garden of the institute run by Katharina Schroth in the 30s in Meissen. [Historical picture from the picture database of Christa Lehnert-Schroth].

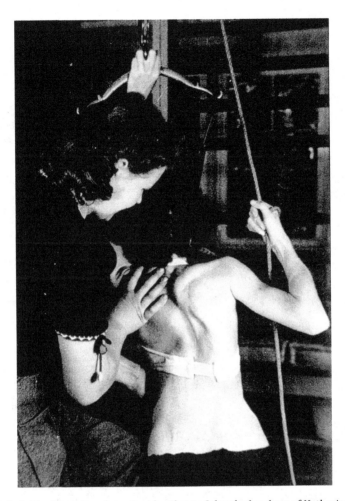

Fig. 2.23: Individual training of a patient by Christa Schroth, daughter of Katharina Schroth, in the 40s. [Historical picture from the picture database of Christa Lehnert-Schroth].

When she began her scoliosis program in Meissen, 1921, (Fig. 2.21 and 2.22) most patients she treated had curvatures exceeding 80° with large rib humps and stiff deformities as a result of scoliosis of varying origins. In the 40s, Christa Schroth (Fig. 2.23) assisted, and helping those with large curves became their main focus (Fig. 2.24 and 2.25).

Besides individual exercises with passive manual correction by a therapist, a group setting was established allowing treatment of patients with similar curve patterns in one group (Fig. 2.26).

The Meissen institute had a large garden and a small building which housed helpful tools for individual and group treatment. When possible, most of the treatment was carried out in the garden. The fresh air and sun's rays contributed to the patients' general health and well-being at a time when people were not used to exposing their skin to the sun or to other people.

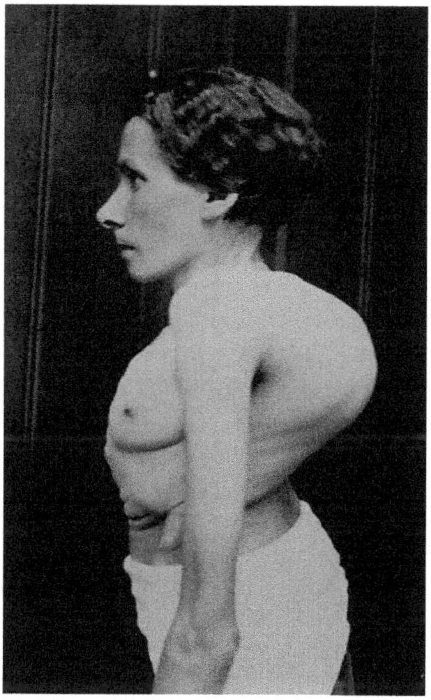

For Katharina Schroth, mirror monitoring was of utmost importance as is demonstrated in Figure 2.17 showing a patient treated by Christa Schroth in the 1940s. Husband and father, Franz Schroth also helped patients in the Meissen institute with individual corrections and special strengthening exercises.

Fig. 2.24: A typical patient with a large curvature as treated in Katharina Schroth's first institute in the 30s in Meissen. [Historical picture from the picture database of Christa Lehnert-Schroth].

It did not take long for controversy to arise and as early as the late 1920s a battle of methods emerged. Professor Scheede from Leipzig, where Hoffa exercises were performed, objected to Katharina Schroth's center mostly because she was neither a professional trainer nor a physician, but had started her program as a school teacher and attended a school of gymnastics after she had started her institute.

After World War II, Katharina Schroth was forced to leave her Meissen institute. She accepted a position of employment to provide her services, with her daughter, now a physical therapist at a state-run medical center in Gottleuba during the early 50s.

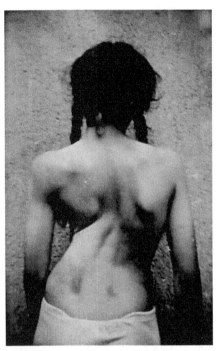

Fig. 2.25: Another typical patient with a large curvature as treated in Katharina Schroth's institute. [Historical picture from the picture database of Christa Lehnert-Schroth, Gottleuba 1950, second Schroth institute, East Germany].

From Gottleuba, Katharina and daughter relocated to Bad Kreuznach, West Germany where they opened a private practice. Christa Schroth married Ernst Weiss, gave birth to a son, Hans-Rudolf Weiss, and divorced. In 1961, mother and daughter established an institute in Sobernheim. This institute attracted many patients, often 150 at a time, with typical stays of six weeks duration (Fig. 2.27 and Fig. 2.28). Christa married Adalbert Lehnert in 1962 who contributed to the growth of this center and was involved in patient treatment.

By the 1970s, Christa Lehnert-Schroth had advanced the method and introduced a simple classification system which is still used today by practitioners (Fig. 2.29). In addition, she discovered the importance of the lumbosacral (counter-) curve (4th curve) for pattern-specific postural correction and described this in her book, *Three-Dimensional Treatment for Scoliosis*, first published in 1973, now available in the 7th English edition (Lehnert-Schroth 2007). This historically important book is available in several languages, including English, Spanish, Mandarin, and Korean.

It was also in the 1970s that a series of investigations were carried out with respect to vital capacity and cardiopulmonary function improvements at the clinic. The findings from these studies resulted in the acknowledgement of the method at some universities (Götze 1976, Götze et al. 1977).

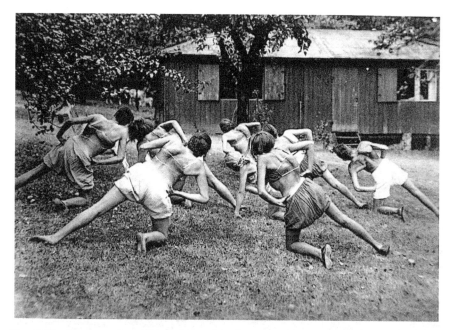

Fig. 2.26: A group of patients with major thoracic curvatures exercising the muscle cylinder. [Historical picture from the picture database of Christa Lehnert-Schroth, Meissen in the 30s].

It was at that same time that the impact of the lumbosacral curve on the correction of certain curve patterns was discovered (Lehnert-Schroth 1981, 1982).

Christa Lehnert-Schroth also recognized the spontaneous correction of a functional leg length discrepancy just by straightening the lumbar curve (Lehnert-Schroth 1981).

It is worth noting that until the end of the 70s, Schroth inpatient practices included passive (cervical) traction, especially for those with large curvatures. This type of treatment was eventually abandoned because of adverse effects. This topic will be discussed further in Chapter 3.

In the early 80s, the Sanatorium Lehnert-Schroth Institute was renamed the Katharina Schroth Clinic, but by this time Katharina Schroth was not as active. Nevertheless, she continued to lobby for her method of treatment having numerous disagreements with professors from various German universities until her death on February 19, 1985.

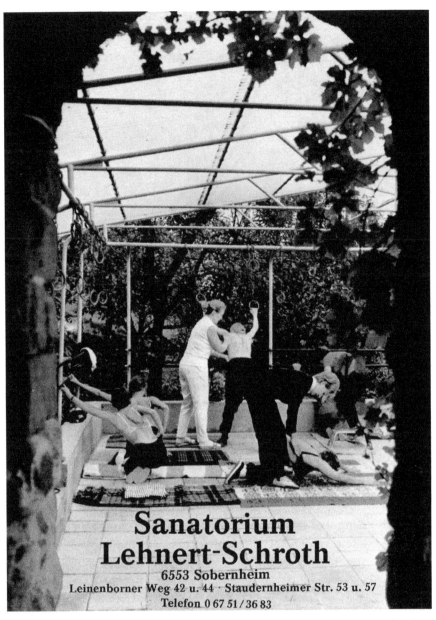

**Sanatorium
Lehnert-Schroth**
6553 Sobernheim
Leinenborner Weg 42 u. 44 · Staudernheimer Str. 53 u. 57
Telefon 0 67 51 / 36 83

Fig. 2.27: Christa Lehnert-Schroth, Katharina Schroth's daughter, amidst a group of patients at her new institute in Sobernheim. (Folder of the Sanatorium Lehnert-Schroth in the 70s). [Historical picture from the picture database of Christa Lehnert-Schroth].

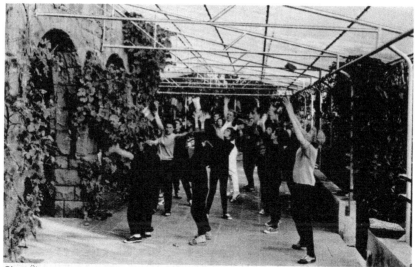

Obere Übungsterrasse

Es wird täglich vor- und nachmittags vielstündig an und mit den Patienten gearbeitet und ihre Eigenverantwortlichkeit geweckt.
Die erste Behandlung sollte mindestens 4-8 Wochen dauern. Vierzehn Tage eignen sich höchstens zur Wiederholung.

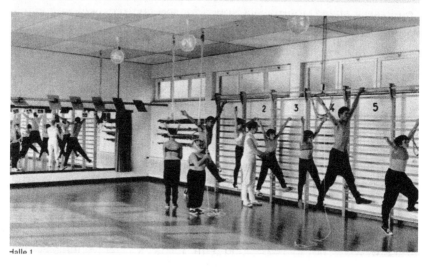

Halle 1

Fig. 2.28: Exercise setting at the Sobernheim institute. (Folder of the Sanatorium Lehnert-Schroth in the 70s). [Historical picture from the picture database of Christa Lehnert-Schroth].

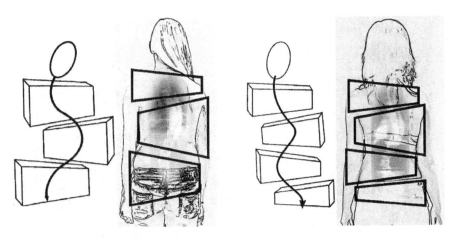

Fig. 2.29: The original classification according to Lehnert-Schroth. On the *left*, the three curve pattern with the shoulder, thoracic, and lumbopelvic block deviated from each other in the frontal plane and also rotated against each other. On the *right*, the four curve pattern with a separation of the lumbopelvic block into a lumbar and a pelvic block deviated from each other in the frontal plane and also rotated against each other. Per definition: the pelvic block symbolizes the lumbosacral counter-curve and this curve is defined as the 4th curve.

First investigations – first scientific evidence

As previously stated, the patient series for the first prospective controlled trial was derived from the patients seen at the clinic from 1989–1991. A sample of results was published in 1995 as a prospective study in German (Weiss 1995). It was published in English for the first time in 1997 (Weiss et al. 1997), and later included age- and sex-matched controls from another regional study on untreated patients as a prospective controlled study (Weiss, Weiss and Petermann 2003). Studies on the improvement of cardiopulmonary capacity, vital capacity improvement, electromyography, and the influence of the treatment of pain were also conducted (Weiss 1991, Weiss 1993a and b, Weiss 1995, Weiss and Bickert 1996, Weiss et al. 1999).

Most of the studies were cohort studies in a pre- / post-intervention design and there were no mid- or long-term follow-ups. Nevertheless, large numbers of patients were studied. Patients (n=794) investigated with ECG showing signs of manifesting right cardiac strain were significantly reduced after an inpatient rehabilitation of six weeks using the Schroth program

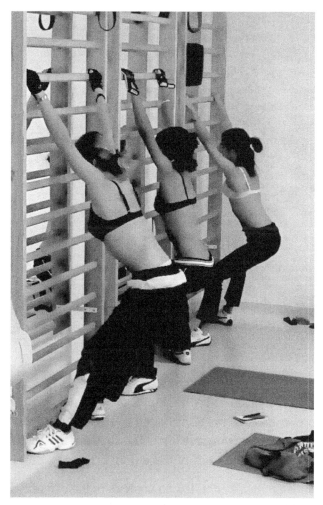

Fig. 2.30: Typical exercise setting in the Katharina Schroth Klinik in Bad Sobernheim. The elevation of both arms leads to an increase of the flat-back deformity [Weiss 2011].

(Weiss and Bickert 1996). More than 800 people were included in a study on vital capacity and rib mobility which was published in *Spine* (Weiss 1991). Another study on muscle activity reductions after intensive rehabilitation consisted of more than 300 patients (Weiss 1993a).

The only mid-term study with a follow-up of more than thirty months was the cohort treated between 1989 and 1991. This study was the basis for a prospective controlled trial published in 2003 (Weiss, Weiss and Petermann 2003).

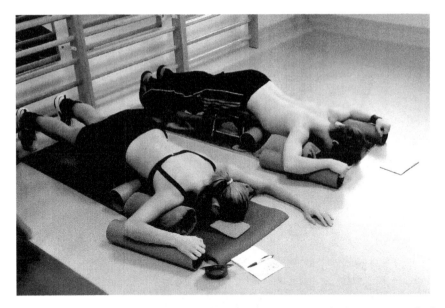

Fig. 2.31: Treatment according to original Schroth instruction methods requires multiple props, not always easily available at home. In this example, because the patient is lying on the floor, they are not able to take advantage of the automated postural correction by using the corrective postural reflex [Weiss 2011].

During the 90s there was development with respect to the correction of thoracolumbar curves including the de-rotational effect of the psoas muscle. More and more exercises were instructed and performed in horizontal positions with numerous corrective tools which were not always easily available for the patient for practice at home (Fig. 2.30 and 2.31).

Previously, the lead author performed an analysis of the different aspects of the original Schroth method (Weiss 1988). One of the most important factors of the original Schroth method is the automated pre-correction of the deformity with the help of postural reflex activity in certain asymmetric upright starting positions. The exercise begins pre-corrected with the help of postural reflex activity in upright asymmetric starting positions and the exercise itself increases this pre-correction.

In horizontal starting positions, these pre-corrections, due to postural reflex activity, cannot be achieved. Therefore the postural corrections cannot be regarded as effective when starting exercise in an asymmetric horizontal position.

Late in the 1980s, Dr. Weiss and his wife initiated a training course for professionals. Dr. Manuel Rigo, an allergist from Spain, was trained as an instructor after a stay in the inpatient Schroth clinic where he learned the basic treatment methods. He then began treating at the clinic bearing the name of his mother-in-law, the Elena Salva Institute in Barcelona. Dr. Rigo then began treating in smaller groups finding success in Spain.

As time passed, however, emphasis was increasingly placed on the correction of pelvic asymmetries in order to address the lumbosacral curve. Unfortunately, the result was that the powerful corrections which initially defined the treatments of Katharina Schroth were being minimized. Corrections were only performed to the midline in order to achieve symmetry, as opposed to overcorrections.

Treatment methodology became more and more complicated, focusing on minute deviations while losing sight of the main curvature correction.

After the Asklepios group took over, the program seemed to become more complex for patients to learn. Unfortunately, it was becoming apparent to the first author, then clinic director, that a clear direction of development was no longer foreseeable and a re-examination of the existing approaches seemed necessary to shift to and focus on more efficient corrective movements.

At that time, the groups of sometimes fifteen to sixteen patients to one therapist were too big for significant patient improvement. The exercise program at the Katharina Schroth Clinic appeared to be stagnant. While the original technique of Katharina Schroth continued to be effective, it seemed to require undue efforts on the part of patients. On the other hand, brace treatment was evolving and improving.

Increasingly, patients with curvature angles of less than 40° and typical flatback deformities were being treated, but there was no real development towards a systematic correction of the sagittal profile.

In marked contrast to that, the original Schroth program was designed for thoracic curves exceeding 80° and trunk rotations and rib humps leading to a more kyphotic inclination of the trunk. Moderate curvatures were addressed quite well in the coronal and transverse planes, but the sagittal profile was not being adequately considered. The only correction of a thoracic flatback was through rotational breathing, while the starting positions of the exercises were still with both arms in elevation, increasing the flatback deformity (Fig. 2.30 and Fig. 2.31).

Schroth/Best Practice goes global

In 2001, coauthor Moramarco contacted Dr. Weiss for advice and treatment of his daughter's scoliosis. Dr. Weiss welcomed the American family to Germany in early 2002 when he was director of the Katharina Schroth Clinic. The authors established an enduring professional relationship. Moramarco continued to pursue study of the original Schroth techniques, including a 2004 course with Rigo and informal training with Christa Lehnert-Schroth, PT.

In 2006, Weiss published his latest developments of newer, more innovative Schroth educational approaches, taking into account the correction of the sagittal profile. (Weiss et al. 2006, Weiss and Klein 2006).

Also in 2006, *Best Practice in Conservative Scoliosis Care* was published. Weiss introduced the principle concepts at the 2007 SOSORT conference in Boston and while there, he invited Dr. Moramarco to Germany for the first international course for Schroth certification where he became the first U.S. Schroth Method practitioner certified at the Asklepios Katharina Schroth Clinic. He returned to establish the first Schroth-based outpatient program using Weiss's cutting edge Scoliologic™ Best Practice treatment protocols, offering patients complete outpatient programs in less than a week.

It is only in the last decade that Schroth methodology has reached beyond the borders of Europe. In the U.S., Moramarco's work with patients incorporates the most innovative evolution of Schroth principles – as do others in the Ukraine, Russia, South Korea and other locales. Dr. Weiss continues to train physicians and therapists internationally as well as focus on continuing improvement of his newest Schroth-compatible brace, the Chêneau-Gensingen®, now offered in North America.

Because patients seek methods to halt progression, improve postural appearance, relieve pain and yearn for alternatives to surgery, the benefits of Schroth-based concepts and bracing are spreading rapidly and are now known and recognized all over the world.

Recent developments

With more than 30,000 evaluations of in-brace x-rays over the past twenty years, the first author has continuously improved not only in-brace corrections, but also the effectiveness of the corrective movements (Weiss and Moramarco 2013).

Since the 2004 add-ons, training times have been shortened, but the concepts are still based on the original three-dimensional treatment approach according to Katharina Schroth.

In 2010, the Schroth Best Practice program was officially established and it is the focus of the remainder of this book. Patients can achieve results within a week, or less, which rivals the previous four to six weeks of inpatient rehabilitation (Weiss and Seibel 2010). Meanwhile, Scoliosis Short-Term Rehabilitation (SSTR) has been tested and the results, as achieved in the pilot investigation, have been shown to be repeatable worldwide (Borysov and Borysov 2012, Pugacheva 2012, Lee 2014).

Physical rehabilitation which focuses on ADLs to avoid loss of postural control during everyday activities is advisable. Add-ons derived from the original Schroth approach aim at unloading the curve and are essential elements for postural control. It is important to note that thirty minutes of scoliosis exercise daily is less effective without knowledge of curve-pattern specific ADLs since without them the curve(s) are loaded during the rest of the day.

It should also be noted that it is important to incorporate physical rehabilitation during brace wear whenever possible, with more intensive work as the patient is weaned from the brace.

The Schroth Best Practice program® has been improved with respect to correction of the sagittal plane. Today, we strive to foster optimal postural correction and here the circle closes again when we consider the remarkable corrections formerly achieved in exceptionally large curvatures.

The newest developments, also referred to as 'New Power Schroth,' as part of the Best Practice program is designed for small, moderate and somewhat severe curvatures. Once a thoracic curve exceeds 70°, the original Schroth program should be incorporated as well to offer the patient the greatest advantage.

Therefore, the newest evolution of Schroth-based therapy (Schroth Best Practice program®) is preferred in curves less than 70° because it is simpler for the patient, addresses the sagittal plane, makes the patient aware of the importance of unloading the spine, and emphasizes the maintenance of postural corrections whenever possible throughout the course of the day.

Reference List

Borysov M, Borysov A. Scoliosis short-term rehabilitation (SSTR) according to 'Best Practice' standards – are the results repeatable? Scoliosis. 2012 Jan 17;7(1):1.

Götze HG. Die Rehabilitation jugendlicher Skoliosepatienten. Untersuchung zur cardiopulmonalen Leistungsfähigkeit und zum Einfluß von Krankengymnastik und Sport. Thesis, Westfälische Wilhelms-Universität, Münster; 1976.

Götze HG, Seibt G, Günther U. Metrische Befunddokumentation pulmonaler Funktionswerte von jugendlichen und erwachsenen Skoliosepatienten unter einer vierwöchigen Kurbehandlung. Z Krankengymnastik. 1977;30:228–233.

Lee SG. Improvement of curvature and deformity in a sample of patients with Idiopathic Scoliosis with specific exercises. OA Musculoskeletal Medicine. 2014; Mar 12;2(1):6.

Lehnert-Schroth C. Unsere Erfahrungen mit einem Verkürzungsausgleich in der Skoliosebehandlung. Orthop Prax. 1981;27:255–262.

Lehnert-Schroth C. Die Beeinflussung der Lumbosakral-Skoliose durch die Dreidimensionale Schroth'sche Skoliosebehandlung. In Die Skoliose, MLV-Gesellschaft, Uelzen Edited by Meznik F, Böhler N. 1982 :116–118.

Lehnert-Schroth C. Three-dimensional treatment for scoliosis. The Martindale Press; 2007.

Oldevig J. Ein neues Gerät und neue Übungen der Schwedischen Heilgymnastik zur Behandlung von Rückgrats-Verkrümmungen. Springer, Berlin; 1913.

Pugacheva N. Corrective exercises in multimodality therapy of idiopathic scoliosis in children - analysis of six weeks efficiency - pilot study. Stud Health Technol Inform. 2012; 176:365-371.

Schroth K. Die Atmungskur. Zimmermann Verlag, Chemnitz; 1924.

Schroth K. Behandlung der Skoliose (Rückgratverkrümmung) durch Atmungsorthopädie. Der Naturarzt. 1931 :11–15.

Schroth K. Wie helfen wir den Rückgratverkrümmten? Obererzgebirgische Zeitung 143, June 25th 1935.

Vasiliadis ES, Grivas TB, Kaspiris A. Historical overview of spinal deformities in ancient Greece. Scoliosis. 2009 Feb 25;4:6.

Weiss HR. Eine funktionsanalytische Betrachtung der dreidimensionalen Skoliosebehandlung nach Schroth. Krankengymnastik. 1988;40:354–363.

Weiss HR. The effect of an exercise program on VC and rib mobility in patients with IS. Spine. 1991;16:88–93.

Weiss HR. Imbalance of electromyographic activity and physical rehabilitation of patients with idiopathic scoliosis. Eur Spine J. 1993a; 1(4):240–243.

Weiss HR. Scoliosis related pain in adult-treatment influences. Eur J Phys Med and Rehab. 1993b;3:91–94.

Weiss HR. The Schroth scoliosis-specific back school—initial results of a prospective followup study. Z Orthop Ihre Grenzgeb. 1995;133:114–117.

Weiss HR, Bickert W. Improvement of the parameters of right-heart stress evidenced by electrocardiographic examinations by the in-patient rehabilitation program according to Schroth in adult patients with scoliosis. Orthop Prax. 1996;32:450–453.

Weiss HR, Lohschmidt K, El Obeidi N, Verres C. Preliminary results and worst-case analysis of inpatient scoliosis rehabilitation. Pedtr Rehabil. 1997 Jan-Mar;1(1):35–40.

Weiss HR, Verres C, El Obeidi N. Ermittlung der Ergebnisqualität der Rehabilitation von Patienten mit Wirbelsäulendeformitäten durch objektive Analyse der Rückenform. Phys Rehab Kur Med. 1999;9:41-47.

Weiss HR, Weiss G, Petermann F. Incidence of curvature progression in idiopathic scoliosis patients treated with scoliosis inpatient rehabilitation (SIR): an age- and sex-matched controlled study. Pediatr Rehabil 2003 Jan-Mar; 6(1):23–30.

Weiss HR, Hollaender M, Klein R. ADL based scoliosis rehabilitation—the key to an improvement of time-efficiency? Stud Health Technol Inform. 2006;123:594–598.

Weiss HR, Klein R. Improving excellence in scoliosis rehabilitation: a controlled study of matched pairs. Pediatr Rehabil. 2006; 9:190–200.

Weiss HR. Best Practice in Conservative Scoliosis Care. 1st edition, Pflaum Munich 2006.

Weiss HR, Seibel S. Scoliosis short-term rehabilitation (SSTR) - a pilot investigation. The Internet Journal of Rehabilitation 2010; 1 Number 1.

Weiss HR, Moramarco M. Scoliosis – treatment indications according to current evidence. OA Musculoskeletal Medicine 2013 Mar 01;1(1):1.

3 Physical rehabilitation specific to scoliosis – a review of the literature

Scoliosis is a three-dimensional deformity of the spine and trunk which may deteriorate quickly during periods of rapid growth (Goldberg et al. 2002, Asher and Burton 2006, Hawes and O'Brien 2006, Weiss and Moramarco 2013). Although scoliosis may be the expression or symptom of certain diseases (e.g., neuromuscular, congenital, or due to certain syndromes or tumors), the majority of patients with scoliosis (80–90%) are idiopathic because the underlying cause has not been determined. Treatment of symptomatic scoliosis may be influenced by the underlying cause. As scoliosis progresses mostly during growth, and in adulthood, the primary goal of intervention is to stop curvature progression (Goldberg et al. 2002, Asher and Burton 2006, Hawes and O'Brien 2006, Weiss and Moramarco 2013).

To understand and interpret the studies on children and adolescents, basic knowledge about growth dynamics may be helpful (Weiss 2012). During childhood and adolescence there are certain times of rapid growth when curvature progression is more probable. During times of slower growth, progression is less likely (Goldberg et al. 2002, Asher and Burton 2006, Hawes and O'Brien 2006) (Fig. 3.1). For example, the "baby spurt" ends at the age of five and a half to six years, followed by a "flat phase" which lasts until the first signs of maturation. Upon the first signs of breast development or pubic hair, the pubertal growth spurt begins (P1) and in its ascending phase (P2-P3), progression may occur (Goldberg et al. 2002). Shortly after the growth peak (P3) – menarche in girls / voice change in boys – the onset of the descending phase of growth occurs until cessation of growth (P5) resulting in skeletal maturity (Weiss 2012).

Curve progression is dependent on growth rate and growth dynamics

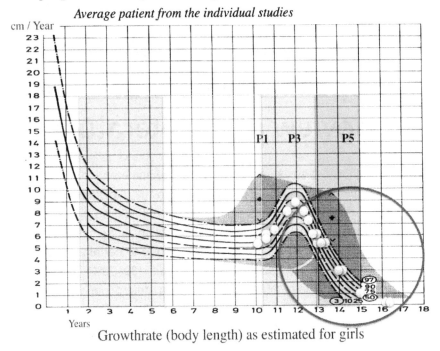

Average patient from the individual studies

Growthrate (body length) as estimated for girls

Fig. 3.1: Growth rate (body length) as estimated for girls. This figure shows that immature individuals experience two phases of growth with higher velocity. One may be called the baby spurt with a descended characteristic (0 to approx. 6 years of age). The other is the pubertal growth spurt (approx. 10 to 13 years). Between these two phases of higher growth velocity, a flat phase of growth with little risk for progression occurs (Figure modified from Weiss and Weiss 2005). The distribution of the average patients from the studies on physiotherapy in scoliosis patients (Weiss 2012) is demonstrated (spots). With kind permission of Pflaum, Munich (Weiss HR: "Best Practice" in Conservative Scoliosis Care, 4th edition, 2012).

In patients with adolescent idiopathic scoliosis (AIS), the risk for progression of Cobb angle (Cobb 1948) can be calculated using a generally accepted progression factor formula (Lonstein and Carlson 1984). Treatment indications for growing adolescents with scoliosis are determined based on this formula (Fig. 3.2). Guidelines derived from this knowledge have been established by SOSORT (Society of Scoliosis Orthopaedic and Rehabilitation Treatment, Weiss et al. 2006) in order to avoid over- and under- treatment.

The formula:

$$\frac{Cobb\ angle - (3 \times Risser\ stage)}{chronological\ age}$$

The product of this formula, the progression factor, may be identified on a correlating chart and can help identify percentage risk of progression (Fig. 3.2). The corresponding estimate can be used as criteria for treatment indications during growth as demonstrated in the international guidelines, included in Chapter 5 (Weiss et al. 2006).

To determine risk of progression, the Risser sign, or epiphyseal growth over the iliac crest (Risser 1958), must be considered. Risser is scaled from 0-5. Premenarcheal girls, on average, are a Risser 0. The Risser sign advances after the onset of menarche for girls and voice change for boys, through skeletal maturity (Risser 5). Risser varies by individual, but clinical experience indicates, generally speaking, that a fourteen-year-old girl usually presents as a Risser 3, sometimes 4, while a fifteen-year-old girl usually presents as a Risser 4, sometimes 5.

Progression factor calculation examples are as follows: a ten-year-old girl with a 20° Cobb angle and a Risser sign of 0 would have a progression factor of 2. The correlating chart indicates a 90% risk of progression. A fifteen-year-old girl with a 20° Cobb angle might typically be 2.6 years postmenarcheal and a Risser 4. When the latter is the case, the progression factor is 0.53 which indicates little risk for progression (Fig. 3.2).

It is important for the practitioner to understand the relationship between potential for growth and risk of progression when considering treatment options, particularly for the patient at high risk. The therapist must know their limitations when considering whether to proceed with physiotherapy alone and its relationship to natural history, considering the lack of existing evidence at this juncture.

A critical review on physiotherapy (Weiss 2012) notes that outcome papers (start of treatment in immature samples/end results after the end of growth; controlled studies in adults with scoliosis with a follow-up of more than five years) were absent in a search of the literature. Some papers investigated mid-term effects of exercises, but most were retrospective. Few were prospective, and many included patient samples with questionable treatment indications.

Moreover, an RCT with measured Cobb angles, comprising a cohort in the progressive phase, with subjects having an indication for physiotherapy (see Chapter 5) and followed from the premenarcheal status until skeletal maturity does not exist. As a matter of fact, many samples noted in the review were mature with little chance of being progressive (Fig. 3.1) with most samples lacking indication for treatment (Fig. 3.2).

Average patient from the individual studies

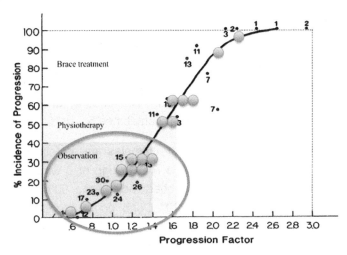

Graph showing the incidence of progression according to the progression factor, which is calculated by the formula:

$$\frac{\text{Cobb angle} - (3 \times \text{Risser stage})}{\text{Chronological age}} = \text{Progression factor}$$

Fig. 3.2: Incidence (risk) of progression can be calculated according to the formula by Lonstein and Carlson (1984). According to the indication guidelines (Weiss et al. 2008) we have to distinguish between an

1. Indication for observation only (Incidence (risk) of progression 40%).
2. Indication for physiotherapy (Incidence (risk) of progression 40–60%).
3. Indication for bracing (Incidence (risk) of progression 60% and more).

The average patient from the majority of papers on physical therapy found have no indication for treatment, but only for observation (spots). With kind permission of Pflaum, Munich (Weiss HR: "Best Practice" in Conservative Scoliosis Care. 4th edition, 2012).

It is not known why scoliosis occurs or why some curves progress and others do not. Roaf (1960) has suggested that spinal imbalance (lateral curvature) leads to asymmetric loading of the vertebral growth plates through gravity and continuous muscle action which then leads to asymmetric growth of the vertebra in accordance with the Hueter-Volkmann principle (Weiss and Hawes 2004).

The mechanism of scoliosis progression during growth has been described by the "vicious cycle" model whereby a scoliosis deformity produces asymmetric loading of the spine. This leads to asymmetric growth, disc and vertebral wedging, and greater deformity (Stokes et al. 2006).

Physical rehabilitation, corrective bracing, and spinal fusion surgery are the treatment modules currently applied in the treatment of scoliosis (Hawes 2003). Physical rehabilitation for scoliosis is by far the under studied, questioned and controversial of the three (Mordecai and Dabke 2012, Romano et al. 2012, Weiss 2012). Historically, surgeons, the gatekeepers of scoliosis treatment, have mostly been opposed to any form of exercise for scoliosis as a form of treatment at any level of risk. Certainly, from the outside looking in, it appears as a group there is little interest in studying how exercise may benefit the scoliosis patient, even if only in terms of creating spinal flexibility for an improved quality of life. Published studies from the U.S. on exercise as it relates to scoliosis are almost nonexistent. In *Scoliosis and the Human Spine*, Hawes notes a long-standing bias against physical rehabilitation for scoliosis in English speaking countries where "watch and wait" is the recommended treatment for mild curves where the resulting lack of early intervention could be perceived as the appearance of a conflict of interest (Hawes 2003).

As mentioned, the scientific literature about physical rehabilitation and scoliosis is scant, especially in comparison to the magnitude of studies regarding surgical techniques or bracing. Recent findings on the current literature supporting physiotherapy conclude that evidence of a higher caliber is needed (Mordecai and Dabke 2012, Weiss 2012). To date, there have been only limited retrospective controlled studies (Level III), a few prospective controlled studies (Level II), and one randomized controlled study (RCT) (Level I) (Weiss 2012). The limited number of studies on exercise efficacy for idiopathic scoliosis have multiple shortcomings (Mordecai and Dabke 2012, Weiss 2012), as previously noted.

One obstacle to such a study would be the limited research or lack of funding for rehabilitative treatment methods by well-funded organizations. The RCT, the gold-standard in research, requires funding and support. The individual practitioner or small organization working to advance specific nonsurgical approaches for those with idiopathic scoliosis would have a difficult time conducting an RCT, or any study requiring a control group for higher level evidence with a large enough sample size. In regard to SRS members, "running a research program and managing a clinical practice essentially are two different professions," (Hawes 2003) and this holds true for the conservative care practitioner as well. Funding from corporations affiliated with surgery for scoliosis, such as the suppliers of $1000 pedicle screws for fusions or the newest hardware for double rod instrumentations, is not a realistic expectation. Corporations whose revenue is based on a function of increasing the number of spinal surgeries, with lengthy fusions, is a reason these entities fund surgeons via consultancies, compensate for advisory positions, and fund research.

For proponents of conservative rehabilitative interventions, perhaps this lack of an RCT better serves the interests of that small subset of adolescent patients who would potentially be randomly assigned to 'watch and wait'. This is based on the premise that education and curve-pattern training are inarguably superior to doing nothing when a scoliosis above 15° exists in an immature patient sample. Beyond that, in accordance with international guidelines (Weiss et al. 2006, guidelines) the pool for such an RCT would be quite limited since any eligible sample would theoretically be restricted to patients having curves between 15° and 19° since indications recommend observation for patients under 15° (Weiss et al. 2006), and bracing for the 'at risk' population, over 20°. In consideration of the recent RCT on bracing (Weinstein et al. 2013), one could claim it is unethical to neglect to brace a progressive curve considering a scoliosis could deteriorate without bracing intervention. Moreover, when larger curves are involved, longer bracing times are required (Weiss 2013) potentially having an enduring impact.

Systematic reviews on the limited published literature, mostly taking place outside the U.S. on exercise rehabilitation are mixed (Fusco et al. 2010, Weiss 2012, Mordecai and Dabke 2012). Of the existing literature, studies have variable designs, many lack controls, follow-up periods are short, assessment methods vary, compliance is questionable, exercise methods are combined with bracing, and adequate statistical analysis is often lacking (Mordecai and Dabke 2012, Weiss 2012). Furthermore, most of the studies considered used patient samples which failed to align with the indications for treatment guidelines. Some studies investigated immature patient samples including curvatures of less than 15°, while the RCT from China included nearly mature patients.

In that RCT (Wan et al. 2005), physical exercise for the treatment of AIS consisted of a patient sample of eighty, with an average age of fifteen ±4 years, with Cobb angles at 24° ±12°. This study could be criticized from a scientific standpoint in that much of the cohort had little risk of progression.

Additionally, the follow-up period was only six months on average. Since, at fifteen years of age, there is usually little *significant* residual growth remaining, the conclusions of this study could be challenged. Although this RCT reported Cobb angle improvement for the treated group, that conclusion is overshadowed considering results could be skewed by spines less at risk for progression due to the mature cohort. One positive is that it did show that physical exercise for scoliosis can be beneficial even at later stages of growth, just prior to bone maturity.

The various international methodologies included in the systematic reviews (Fusco et al. 2010, Mordecai and Dabke 2012, Weiss 2012) critique studies on the various exercise approaches. Most of consequences are referenced at the end of this chapter for the interested reader.

Maruyama et al. (2003) showed that treatment of curves in the 20°-40° range respond more favorably in comparison to curves on the threshold of surgery. This point strengthens the case for earlier intervention via exercise instruction. An important point remains; no studies, of any nature, of any size, exist for AIS comparing a treated to an untreated control group with subjects having curvatures of moderate magnitude or greater.

Glassman evaluates conservative treatment of adult scoliosis patients (Glassman et al. 2010). Two others studied operative versus nonoperative treatment (Bridwell et al. 2009, Li et al. 2009). It is important to distinguish the difference. Nonoperative does not imply, indicate or necessarily include curve pattern-specific scoliosis exercise rehabilitation.

In the study on adults undergoing 'conservative' treatments, the modalities included were defined as medication, unspecified exercise therapy, general physical therapy modalities (e.g., electrical muscle stimulation), injections/blocks, chiropractic, bracing, and bedrest. This study questioned the value of nonsurgical treatment for adults with scoliosis, concluding that documented costs are "substantial" with no improvement in health status observed for two years (Glassman et al. 2010). These conclusions were based on a study combining several methods, and deem nonsurgical treatment, as a whole, ineffective and costly without including any specific exercise-based approach. Limitations were acknowledged, but conclusions were drawn in spite of the admitted shortcomings, "An important caveat of this study was that the treatment was not randomized and therefore the treatment group might have deteriorated if not for the treatment they received."

At this juncture, it is probably clear that research into conservative therapeutic methods for scoliosis is not comparable, lacks substantive follow-up and drawing conclusions from a scientific standpoint about exercise approaches for scoliosis is challenging, at best, from the mixed body of evidence (Fusco et al. 2010, Weiss 2012, Mordecai and Dabke 2012).

However, practitioners committed to advancing exercise rehabilitation continue to persevere and improve treatment standards for patients and families that feel quite alone at times in terms of their best interests or options for treatment. For this reason, the body of evidence will continue to grow. A new RCT, recently published, is promising and adds to the limited body of evidence. This new Level I study focuses on self-correction (autocorrection) and task-oriented movements to reduce curvature (Monticone et al. 2014).

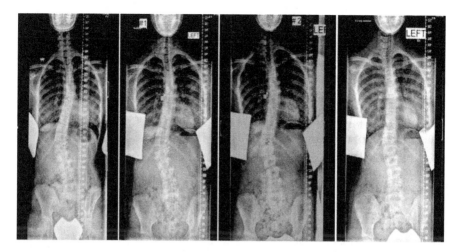

Fig. 3.3: This fourteen-year-old patient, never braced, participated in the first Schroth Best Practice Program in the U.S. in July, 2008. Initial Cobb angles: *(Left)* 6/2008 at 26° left thoracic (T5-T10) and right thoracolumbar at 41° (T10-L3). *Left Center (LC), Right Center* (RC) and *Right* (R) x-ray images taken on 1/2009. (LC) 22°/37°, (RC) elongation at 21°/30°, and (R) with side-shift (translation) and elongation 18°/22°. 7/2008 ATR°: 7° thoracic/13° thoracolumbar. Five years later, 2/2014 ATR°: 4° thoracic/9° thoracolumbar. (X-ray with permission from Dr. Marc Moramarco, Scoliosis 3DC™, Woburn, MA).

Schroth methodology and Best Practice®

The authors' experience collectively comprises more than a century dedicated to delivering the most highly evolved scoliosis-specific rehabilitative technique in existence. The Schroth method scoliosis-specific treatment has helped improve the lives of scoliotics, now internationally, and provides the compliant patient the opportunity to affect curvature. Results often include halted progression in adults and/or Cobb angle improvement in adolescents (Weiss, Weiss and Petermann 2003, Otman 2005, Lehnert-Schroth 2007; Fig. 3.3), improved postural appearance (Lehnert-Schroth 2007), improved muscular imbalance (Weiss 1993a), reduction or elimination of pain (Weiss 1993b), and improved vital capacity and chest expansion (Weiss 1991).

Research in support of Schroth-based therapies based on three-dimensional correction include Schroth method inpatient investigations dating back to 1991. A study published in *Spine*, (Weiss 1991) determined that the Schroth method improved vital capacity and rib mobility in a cohort from the Katharina Schroth Clinic inpatient program. Other documented benefits have been that the Schroth method improves quality of life and the self-concept of scoliosis patients (Weiss and Cherdron 1992, 1994), there is a beneficial effect on muscular imbalance (Weiss 1993a) and pain (Weiss 1993b), and another study showed a Schroth program may enable the reduction of right cardiac strain after intensive scoliosis-specific exercise (Weiss and Bickert 1996).

A Saudi Medical Journal published an independent Schroth study from Turkey providing additional evidential reinforcement that curve-pattern specific exercise can have a beneficial influence on the clinical signs and symptoms of scoliosis. The study concluded that Schroth breathing and exercise can positively influence Cobb angle, vital capacity, muscle strength and postural defects in adolescents participating in an outpatient program (Otman et al. 2005). Most notably, after six weeks Cobb angles decreased over time, with Cobb angle improvements exceeding the 5° margin of error (Morrissy et al. 1990), the accepted benchmark to document change. Vital capacities increased, providing long-term validation of Schroth method improvement of lung function (Weiss 1991). The Otman et al. study reported Cobb angle improvement in all but one subject who experienced stabilization. None worsened, and after one year each patient experienced improvement to some degree.

Added evidence from a prospective controlled study comparing Schroth treated patients versus untreated control groups during growth show a percentage were stablized. In addition, when comparing the untreated control group to an inpatient treated group consisting of the most severe curves, there was a significant difference in terms of reduction of incidence of curve progression in the treated group (Weiss, Weiss and Petermann 2003).

As a result of these recent findings, Schroth Best Practice® is the newest evolution of the Schroth method. During Best Practice® instruction, the patient is taught to achieve optimal postural control during daily activities by incorporating 3-D corrective movements into every day life. These newest concepts allow efficiency (Weiss and Klein 2006) combining more modern, effective and simpler techniques with Schroth methodology in the outpatient setting. This helps the patient achieve heightened postural awareness via active self-correction techniques. These newest methods are essential to stimulate stabilization and encourage balance in the scoliotic spine (Monticone 2014).

The Schroth Best Practice program combines several components for the treatment of scoliosis, including self-correction. According to SOSORT, autocorrection is considered the key technique when physical exercise is utilized for scoliosis rehabilitative techniques (Fusco et al. 2010). The recent RCT validates the effectiveness of self-correction (Monticone et al. 2014). Since the Best Practice methodology combines autocorrection with Schroth principles, it offers patients a new, more viable rehabilitative approach via exercise because postural correction plays a major role in exercise rehabilitation, as it does in bracing (Landauer et al. 2003).

Self-correction maneuvers are important for the scoliotic and essential for constructing that corrected sense of posture. It is only via asymmetric trunk muscle tension that the corrected posture can be easily perceived. This is best achieved in the upright position to trigger postural reflex activity (activation of the segmental spinal muscles). 3-D self-correction is an essential preliminary for effective Schroth exercise since the pelvis is recompensated, any thoracic or lumbar rib humps are addressed and the sagittal profile is restored.

The recent Schroth Best Practice developments (Weiss, Hollaender and Klein 2006, Weiss and Klein 2006) also incorporate side-shift as part of the protocol. When performing self-correction, side-shift (translation) plays a role. Side-shift maneuvers help to accomplish the needed translation and are exercise maneuvers which potentially result in a reduction of curvature of up to 10° in some patients (Maruyama et al. 2002). Additional findings have shown that progression may be slowed in the skeletally mature scoliotic when side-shift and hitch exercises are incorporated daily (Maruyama et al. 2002).

Translation movements are favorable for scoliotic curves under 50° (White and Panjabi 1976) and support the asymmetric autocorrections performed in the frontal plane and are superior to elongation (traction) for postural correction. Elongation in a biomechanical model is superior to translation for curves greater than 50° (White and Panjabi 1976), but in practice, a combination of these particular maneuvers may be effective, regardless of the curvature degree.

Physio-logic® exercises address scoliosis in the sagittal profile and are also an important component of the Best Practice protocols. It is important to address the sagital profile (van Loon 2008, Monticone 2014). The physio-logic® exercises were studied in a pilot program (Weiss and Seibel 2010) incorporating the add-ons to scoliosis rehabiliation. The physio-logic® technique created reduced lateral deviation of the scoliotic trunk (Weiss and Klein 2006).

When progressive sagittal imbalance occurs, curve severity increases in a linear fashion (Glassman et al. 2005). Kyphosis is more favorable in the upper thoracic region, but poorly tolerated in the lumbar spine. Evidence shows that scoliosis correction in the sagittal plane leads to a 3-D correction of the curves in an experimental (Weiss 2005) and clinical study (Weiss and Klein 2006). During physical rehabilitation via exercises derived from the original Schroth program, and bracing techniques that align with Schroth principles, efforts of focus are on correcting the sagittal alignment to restore lumbar lordosis and thoracic kyphosis (Weiss 2011).

During a two-week program, this ADL approach combining side-shift, physio-logic®, and 3D-ADL exercises with Schroth-based exercises resulted in similar improvements of lateral deviation and trunk rotation when compared to the traditional four-week inpatient program of Schroth based exercise. These developments offer a time-efficiency of treatment for the scoliotic (Weiss, Hollaender and Klein 2006).

Another component, the signature of Schroth, is rotatory breathing, the technique responsible for the longevity and success of the original Schroth inpatient program. In combination with the newer modifications of the Schroth Best Practice® outpatient program, patients can now work to improve vital capacity and rib mobility with the added benefit of incorporating techniques into everyday living.

The new Schroth developments (Schroth Best Practice program®) have spread internationally into the U.S., Canada, Ukraine, Russia, China, Hong Kong, Taiwan and Korea. In the Ukraine, documented improvement of ATR the thoracic convex side dorsally, due to the counter-rotation. These statements refer to the spatial position of the pelvis, taking into account a patient-oriented coordination system. For this, we use the terms "geometric" and "spatial pelvic torsion." In contrast, the one-sided elongation of the intrinsically lumbar portion of the autochthonic back musculature, as well as the sacroiliac joint mechanism, produce an anteversion of the wing of the ilium on the thoracic convex side (on this side the transverse processes of the lumbar spine are rotated away from the iliac crest in the ventral direction which distances the origin and approach of the intrinsic lumbar musculature from each other).

Due to the static alterations described, incorrect pelvic positioning has an impact on the coxofemoral joint connection in the case of a functional 4-curve scoliosis: the hip joint on the thoracic concave side therefore experiences relative abduction, rotation outwards, and extension, while the lower part of the leg from the knee downwards is more likely to rotate inward.

The altered pelvic geometry has an unfavorable impact on the symmetry of the anatomic reference points of the lower extremities.

For functional 4-curve scoliosis, Lehnert-Schroth (1981) established a typical asymmetry in the position of the anterior superior iliac spines (ASIS). On the thoracic concave side, the anterior iliac spines stand in a ventrocaudal relation to the thoracic convex side. The anterior iliac spines on the thoracic convex side stand in more of a dorsocranial relation.

With functional 4-curve curvatures, it is usually a case of lumbar or thoracolumbar scoliosis, and these are sometimes larger and stiffer than the thoracic equalization curvatures. With this curvature pattern we may see a decompensation of the trunk toward the thoracic concave side, hip prominence on the thoracic convex side, and an increased strain on the leg on the thoracic concave side.

6.1.6 Typical features of the 4CL pattern (Fig. 6.17, 6.18)

The 4CL pattern (functional 4-curve, lumbar or functional 4-curve with singular lumbar curvature) is characterized by the existence of a lumbar major curvature with the appropriate cranial and caudal equalization curvatures. A lumbosacral countercurve can be identified radiologically via the wedge-shaped intervertebral spaces L4–S1. The thoracic secondary curvature is only slightly visible and the cervicothoracic equalization curvature usually is not visible with this pattern. This pattern is normally decompensated in the lumbar convex region (weak side). One can identify the typical hip prominence on the parcel side, which is an approach for the correction maneuver.

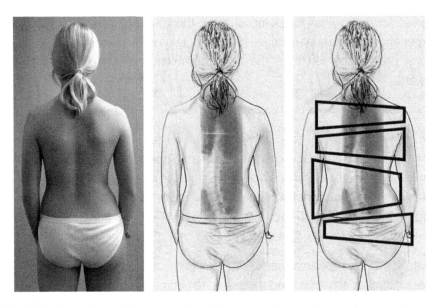

Fig. 6.17: The pattern 4CL, or functional 4-curve with singular lumbar curvature, is characterized by the fact that a single major curvature exists, with the appropriate cranial and caudal equalization curvatures. The thoracic secondary curvature appears only slightly and the cervicothoracic equalization curvature is even less visible. This pattern is usually decompensated in the lumbar region. In the *middle*, the silhouette of the trunk is shown with an x-ray overlay. On the *right*, the trunk wedge, which, for the sake of clarity, has not been shown three-dimensionally. Note: the prominent trunk parts, characterized by the thick end of the wedge, are always twisted in a dorsal direction.

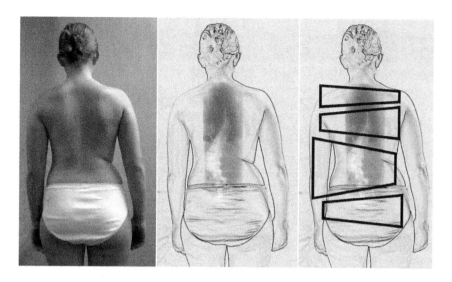

Fig. 6.18: A further example of pattern 4CL. In the *middle*, the silhouette of the trunk is shown with an x-ray overlay. On the *right*, the trunk wedge, which, for the sake of clarity, has not been shown three-dimensionally. Note: the prominent trunk parts, characterized by the thick end of the wedge, are always twisted in a dorsal direction.

6.1.7 Typical features of the 4CTL pattern (Fig. 6.19)

The pattern 4CTL (functional 4-curve, thoracolumbar) or functional 4-curve with singular thoracolumbar curvature is characterized by a thoracolumbar major curvature with the according cranial and caudal equalization curvatures. With the 4CTL pattern, the apical vertebra usually is L1. In rare cases (Fig. 6.20) the apex can also lie with T12/L1. An apical vertebra at T12 would be reason to opt for pattern 3CTL (compare Fig. 6.12). A lumbosacral countercurve is by definition detectable radiologically, due to the wedge-shaped intervertebral spaces L4–S1. The thoracic secondary curvature is only slightly visible and the cervicothoracic equalization curvature usually is not visible with this pattern. This pattern is decompensated in the lumbar region (to the weak side). One can see the typical hip prominence on the parcel side, which is an approach for the correction maneuver.

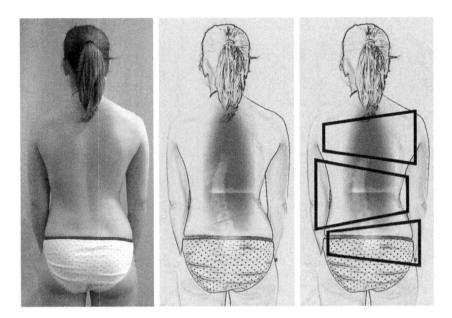

Fig. 6.19: The pattern 4CTL, or functional 4-curve with singular thoracolumbar curvature is characterized by the existence of a thoracolumbar major curvature (apical vertebra L1), with the appropriate cranial and caudal equalization curvatures. The thoracic secondary curvature appears only slightly and the cervicothoracic equalization curvature is even less visible. This pattern is normally decompensated in the lumbar region (or in the thoracolumbar region). In the *middle*, the silhouette of the trunk is shown with an x-ray overlay. On the *right*, the trunk wedge, which, for the sake of clarity, has not been shown three-dimensionally. Note: the prominent trunk parts, characterized by the thick end of the wedge, are always twisted in a dorsal direction.

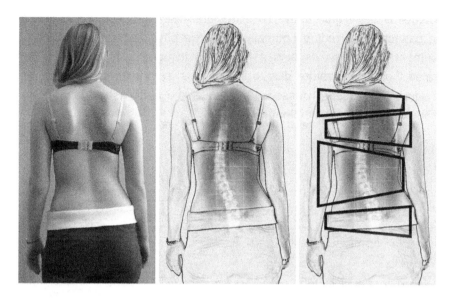

Fig. 6.20: A further example of pattern 4CTL. With this curvature the apex of the curvature is located in the intervertebral space at T12/L1. In the *middle*, the silhouette of the trunk is shown with an x-ray overlay. On the *right*, the trunk wedge, which, for the sake of clarity, has not been shown three-dimensionally. Note: the prominent trunk parts, characterized by the thick end of the wedge, are always twisted in a dorsal direction.

6.1.8 Typical features of a structural double-thoracic scoliosis (Fig. 6.21)

There are more patterns of curvature than have been presented. Some of them appear so infrequently that they cannot be systematically treated, but must be approached individually. However, double thoracic scoliosis is very common and should be mentioned as a special case. Double thoracic curves can be classified either as a functional 3-curve or a functional 4-curve, and can appear along with all functional 3-curve patterns, and more rarely with the 4C pattern.

The double thoracic scoliosis can appear of its own accord or as a complication of brace treatment. It is characterized by the fact that the cervicothoracic equalization curve is structurally changed resulting in the appearance of a so-called "shoulder hump" on the weak side. The shoulder on the weak side sits high, and radiologically one can observe a T1 tilt to the parcel side (Definition King V). This pattern is usually not decompensated significantly. The structural cervicothoracic curve is short and cannot be corrected optimally either via physiotherapy or with brace treatment. This curve is also a hindrance to correction for the caudally located thoracic curvature due to its stiffness. A structural cervicothoracic curvature can appear in association with all the patterns described above which exhibit a thoracic major curvature.

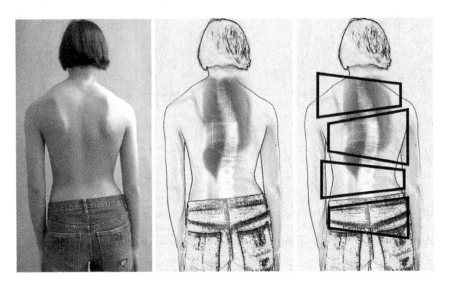

Fig. 6.21: Double thoracic scoliosis is characterized by the fact that the cervicothoracic equalization curve is structurally altered and a "shoulder hump" has evolved. The shoulder on the weak side sits higher, and radiographically, the T1 vertebra is tilted to the parcel side (Definition King V). This pattern is usually not particularly decompensated. In the *middle*, the silhouette of the trunk is shown with an x-ray overlay. On the *right*, the trunk wedge, which, for the sake of clarity, has not been shown three-dimensionally. Note: the prominent trunk parts, characterized by the thick end of the wedge, are always twisted in a dorsal direction.

Reference List

Asher MA, Burton DC. Adolescent idiopathic scoliosis: natural history and long-term treatment effects. Scoliosis. 2006;1(1):2.

Burwell RG. Aetiology of idiopathic scoliosis: current concepts. Pediatr Rehabil. 2003 Jul-Dec;6(3-4):137-70.

Dickson RA, Lawton JO, Archer IA, Butt WP. The pathogenesis of idiopathic scoliosis. Biplanar spinal asymmetry. J Bone Joint Surg Br. 1984 Jan;66(1):8–15.

King HA. Selection of fusion levels for posterior instrumentation and fusion in idiopathic scoliosis. Orthop Clin North Am. 1988 Apr;19(2):247–255.

Lehnert-Schroth C. Unsere Erfahrungen mit einem Verkürzungsausgleich in der Skoliosebehandlung. Orthop Prax. 1981;27:255–262.

Lehnert-Schroth C. Three-dimensional treatment for scoliosis. The Martindale Press; 2007.

Lenke LG, Betz RR, Bridwell KH, Clements DH, Harms J, Lowe TG, Shufflebarger HL. Intraobserver and interobserver reliability of the classification of thoracic adolescent idiopathic scoliosis. J Bone Joint Surg Am. 1998 Aug;80(8):1097–1106.

Lenke LG. Lenke classification system of adolescent idiopathic scoliosis: treatment recommendations. Instr Course Lect. 2005;54:537–542.

Rigo M. Intraobserver reliability of a new classification correlating with brace treatment. Pediatric Rehabilitation. 2004;7:63.

Rigo MD, Villagrasa M, Gallo D. A specific scoliosis classification correlating with brace treatment: description and reliability. Scoliosis. 2010 Jan 27;5(1):1. doi: 10.1186/1748-7161-5-1.

Tomaschewski R. Die Frühbehandlung der beginnenden idiopathischen Skoliose. In: Weiss, H.R.: Wirbelsäulendeformitäten (Vol. 2), Gustav Fischer Verlag, Stuttgart, 51–58, 1992.

van Loon PJ, Kühbauch BA, Thunnissen FB. Forced lordosis on the thoracolumbar junction can correct coronal plane deformity in adolescents with double major curve pattern idiopathic scoliosis. Spine. 2008 Apr 1;33(7):797–801.

Weiss HR. "Brace technology" thematic series - the Gensingen brace™ in the treatment of scoliosis. Scoliosis. 2010 Oct 13;5:22.

Weiss HR, Moramarco M. Scoliosis – treatment indications according to current evidence. OA Musculoskeletal Medicine 2013 Mar 01;1(1).

7 The Schroth Scoliologic® 'Best Practice' Program

In 2006, after the completion of the second edition of this book, the first edition of the book *"Best Practice" in Conservative Scoliosis Care* was published by Pflaum Press. The fourth edition became available in 2012 and contains a brief description of the program detailed here (Weiss 2012).

The Schroth-based Scoliologic® Best Practice program has been under development since 2004, and its individual components have been undergoing scientific testing since 2006 (Weiss and Klein 2006, Weiss, Hollaender and Klein 2006). In the process, it has been determined that the sagittal configuration must be improved to optimize the results of the traditional Schroth method of treatment. Furthermore, a prospective and controlled study showed that scoliosis rehabilitation can occur over shorter periods with these updated techniques, with particular consideration given to everyday activities (Weiss, Hollaender and Klein 2006).

The developments introduced following these new insights are now the foundation of the most efficient and effective short-term rehabilitation programs offered via outpatient services, or scoliosis-specific back schools (Weiss and Seibel 2010, Borysov and Borysov 2012, Pugacheva 2012, Lee 2014). In bracing, and via rehabilitation through optimal educational programs, practitioners instruct patients seeking ways to minimize the extent to which quality of life for those with scoliosis is compromised.

Currently, outpatient concepts of rehabilitation have similar results to inpatient intensive rehabilitation (SIR), at least in terms of the surgical incidence (Maruyama 2003, Weiss, Reiter and Rigo 2003). The results of inpatient intensive rehabilitation are based on collectives of patients treated for six-week intervals from the 1980s to the beginning of the 1990s (Weiss, Weiss and Petermann 2003).

According to a recent review, there are no results for the recent significantly modified contemporary concepts of inpatient scoliosis rehabilitation with reduced rehabilitation time (Yilmaz and Kozikoglu 2010). Consequently, the step to short-term outpatient rehabilitation is justified.

The Schroth Best Practice Program® contains the following components:
- The physio-logic® program for correction of the sagittal profile
- Education related to everyday activities (ADLs)
- The program "3D made easy"
- The new "Power Schroth" program

Use of the treatment techniques mentioned are described below.

7.1 The physio-logic® program

Several authors have concluded that thoracic flatback can promote thoracic idiopathic scoliosis (Deacon and Flood 1984, Tomaschewski 1987, Weiss and Lauf 1995, Burwell 2003, Raso 2000) (Fig. 7.1–7.2), as Farkas did in 1925. If the rotation and the lateral deviation of the spine are secondary characteristic patterns of idiopathic scoliosis, then it should be possible to correct or improve the three-dimensional deformity of scoliosis solely through the application of sagittal movements of force.

Flatback is a larger problem, at least with brace provision for patients with idiopathic scoliosis. Articles have been published showing that flatback can actually be increased by certain bracing concepts. For example, pressure zones for correcting the sagittal profile are not found on either the Boston brace or the Charleston bending brace, nor on most other types of braces. It was not until the original Chêneau brace that pressure zones for the correction of a thoracic hypokyphosis were introduced (Weiss and Moramarco 2013).

Until now, therapeutic treatment programs have primarily focused on the frontal plane deformity (Klapp 1907, von Niederhöffer 1942, Ocarzuk 1994); few programs set the correction of the spinal rotation as a target (Rigo et al. 1991, Klisic and Nikolic 1985, Mollon and Rodot 1986, Lehnert-Schroth 2007). The sagittal profile has been of less interest in physiotherapeutic approaches (Tomaschewski 1992, Weiss and Moramarco 2013). Prior to

1992, Antonio Negrini pointed out that the sagittal profile should be restored using correctional exercises (Negrini 1992). In some exercise programs, flatback is of central importance; however, no favorable results were achieved with general kyphosing exercises (Ducongé 1992). All patients treated via a program that "hyperkyphosized" the entire trunk (global kyphosis) experienced a worsening of their condition within a year of dedicated treatment. Due to this latter study, it can be concluded that it is not sensible to mobilize the spine in the direction of a global kyphosis.

With the Schroth program, one tries to restore the thoracic kyphosis using a special breathing technique, in conjunction with special exercises that have a thoracic kyphosis-inducing effect.

There is recent evidence indicating that the corrective forces operating in the sagittal plane can also

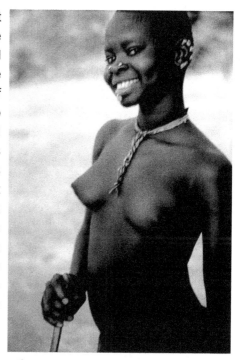

Fig. 7.1: With primitive people, a "forward placement" of the trunk can often be observed and for this reason be seen as natural and "sensible" (Photo © LRP, published in Weiss HR, Weiss G. Physiologic balance® - the simple and relaxed way to a healthy back. Pflaum, Munich, 2013). This trunk attitude, with an increased lumbar lordosis, leads to a lateral stabilization, which can also straighten out spinal distortions (van Loon et al. 2008).

correct scoliotic deformity in the transverse and frontal planes (van Loon et al. 2008). An experimental study with the goal of using surface measurement to document the short-term corrective effect of two different braces showed that sagittal corrective forces can lead to similar short-term corrections as those from the three-dimensional correctional forces that operate with the Chêneau brace (Weiss et al. 2006).

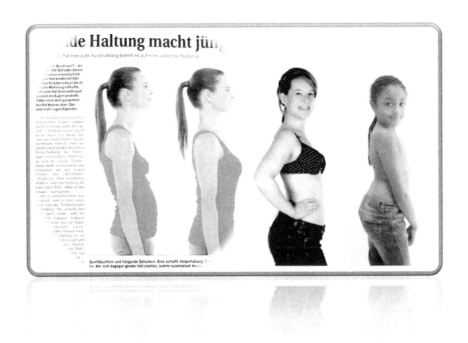

Fig. 7.2: *Left:* From the service pages of our newspaper (Public Gazette Nr. 182 – 8.8.2009): "Sticking-out stomach and hanging shoulders: droopy posture (*left*) isn't attractive. Someone who carries themselves properly (*middle left*) automatically makes a better impression." The posture on the *far left* is certainly not desirable! The "upright posture" shown looks more like the woman has swallowed a metal pole. In our opinion, the two women on the *right* make the best impression (*middle right*, optimal natural posture and *far right* an eight-year-old with her natural, strong posture).

If the Lehnert-Schroth three-dimensional scoliosis treatment can achieve long-term changes for a scoliosis patient (Lehnert-Schroth 2007), then the results of the aforementioned study indicates that the quality of physiotherapeutic scoliosis rehabilitation can be improved through adding increased corrections in the sagittal plane. Working with this foundation, an exercise program with the aim of restoring a physiological sagittal profile (Fig. 7.3–7.4) has been developed. These exercises have the same basic principles, namely, strengthening and improving the lordosis at the level of L2, as well as strengthening and improving the thoracic kyphosis in the mid-thoracic region (Fig. 7.1 and 7.2, Fig. 7.5).

These exercises are the physio-logic® exercises. The results achieved in a study with matched age, sex, pattern of curvature, and Cobb angle concur with the hypothesis that through the application of physio-logic® exercises, one can improve the treatment results of scoliosis (Weiss and Klein 2006).

There are indications that the preservation of the lumbar lordosis in adulthood is of paramount importance. Glassman et al. (2005) discovered that the sagittal profile has a decisive influence on the stability of a scoliosis. Also, van Loon, Kühbauch, and Thunnissen (2008) have shown that restoration of the lumbar lordosis leads to correction of the spinal curvature in patients with scoliosis. Taking this into account, it is now scientifically accepted that the "relordosation" of the lumbar spine is important for the correction of scoliosis and its stabilization.

7.1.1 Description of the physio-logic® exercise program

The physio-logic® exercise program consists of the following:
- symmetric mobilization exercises for improving the lordosis with a target course of L1/2 and mobilizing the kyphosis of the lower thoracic spine
- education regarding the physio-logic® approach for everyday activities.

The symmetric mobilization exercises are done repeatedly. These exercises can only be performed with the help of passive resistance or with the help of postural reflexes. With the physio-logic® exercises, the focus is on increasing the lumbar lordosis while simultaneously channeling force into the kyphosis of the lower thoracic spine. When standing, the lumbar lordosis can be increased by tilting the pelvis (with the upper part of the trunk flexed slightly backwards against the lordosis). This starting position improves the kyphosis of the thoracic spine reflectively, a correction maneuver that is desirable with idiopathic thoracic scoliosis. However, the aim of this exercise is not to increase the lumbar lordosis at the L5/S1 level, since this could trigger back pain. Instead, the lordosis should have its apex at the level of L2 or at the intervertebral disc level L1/L2. This can be ensured if both lower costal arches are brought forward (Weiss and Klein 2006). When performed optimally, a trunk position that is corrected in this way requires no noticeable muscular tension (Fig. 7.3).

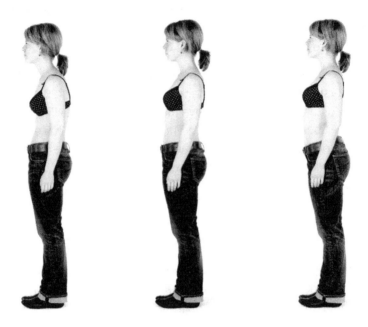

Fig. 7.3: When tensing the stomach muscles in an upright standing position, the upper trunk and shoulders automatically move forward (*left*). In order to remain upright, the shoulders must be held back actively (*middle*). This causes constant tightness, decreased blood circulation, and painful tension. If one brings the front costal arches further forward (see Fig. 7.1), the hollow curve in the upper lumbar region is increased, the upper body can balance itself better, the shoulders slide more loosely backwards, and the muscular tension needed to stand upright is barely noticeable.

For the asymmetric three-dimensional correction of posture, we take the Schroth exercises and modify them according to the principles of the physio-logic® program. Tilting the pelvis and ventralization of the lower costal arch replace the first and second pelvic corrections from the original Schroth program.

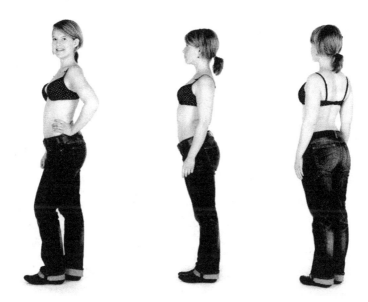

Fig. 7.4: In order to learn the moves the posture correction is exaggerated. Since it is usually a lifestyle with too much sitting that must be compensated for, the upper lumbar spine must become accustomed to the possibility of correction. Contractions must be eliminated so that the correction function can be carried out.

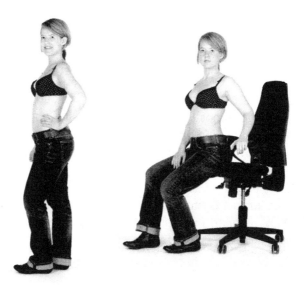

Fig. 7.5: Everyday posture from the physio-logic® program in standing and seated positions.

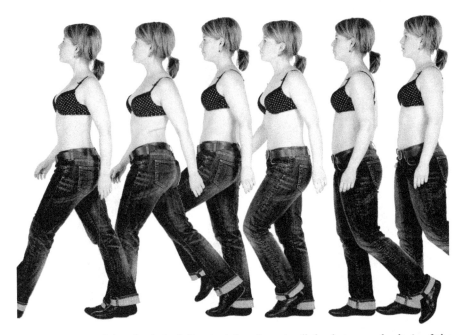

Fig 7.6: As part of the physio-logic® principles, the catwalk leads to a re-lordosis of the upper lumbar spine and to a re-kyphosis in the chest region. While walking, the lower costal arches should seesaw forward. In daily life, this exercise can be carried out very inconspicuously. Ideally, the physio-logic® program exercises should all be carried out with the trunk leaning slightly forward.

The catwalk physio-logic® has two phases: 1. The unrolling phase (placing of the heel to the placing of the sole). 2. The free leg phase (placing of the toes to the removal of the foot from the ground). With phase 1 (*left*), the lumbar hollow curve is maximized; with phase 2 (3rd image from the *right*) it is reduced. Left (1), middle (2), right (1) other leg.

Everyday activities (ADL training) are of the utmost importance to effect change in the habitual posture. For this reason, the physio-logic® everyday training program is carried out in a standing position and while walking as well (Fig. 7.4–7.6). In addition, patients also learn the catwalk, which contains the basic principles of the physio-logic® program just as the 'NUBA' posture (Fig. 7.1) does as a starting point. This position descended from the physiological posture of members from a North African tribe that live in a natural manner. Further exercises from the physio-logic® program are represented in Figures 7.7, Figure 7.8, and Figure 7.9.

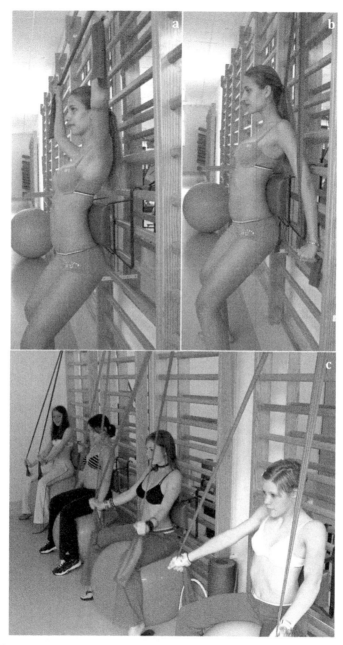

Fig. 7.7: The exercise "snake on the ledge" can be carried out either standing **(a,b)** or sitting **(c)**. With it we achieve passive counter-support of the lumbar lordosis and mobilize the thoracic spine by using kyphosis-inducing synergy effects via pulling the arms downward against the resistance of an elastic band, going into inner rotation/abduction.

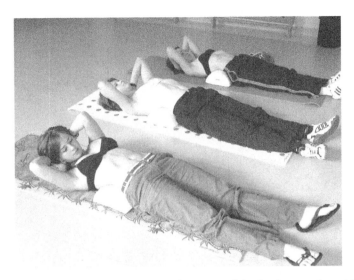

Fig. 7.8: A passive counter-support of the lumbar spine while simultaneously mobilizing the thoracic spine into the kyphosis. In this exercise, the upper trunk should not be elevated to the extent that the contact between the lumbar spine and the cushion lying underneath is separated.

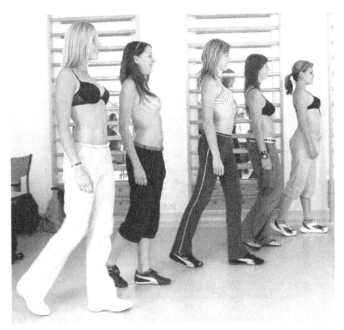

Fig. 7.9: The catwalk, used here with a group of patients, takes the physio-logic® principles into consideration.

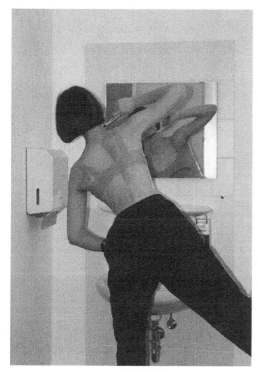

Fig. 7.10: A patient brushing her teeth in the morning in the "muscle cylinder" starting position.

7.2 Instruction in everyday activities (ADL)

Utilizing Schroth exercises in everyday situations can be a decisive factor in generating motivation, and the exercises are more easily performed than strict exercises with a defined starting position. However, concern is not only with integrating exercises in everyday situations (the muscle cylinder can easily be carried out while cleaning your teeth, see Fig. 7.10), but also so the patient learns positions of rest where the spine can be put in a corrective position to decrease the asymmetric loading on the vertebral bodies and intervertebral discs.

It is usually more comfortable to rest in a curved position as defined by a scoliotic curve. This is, therefore, a hurdle that the patient must overcome. The practitioner shows the patient how to become comfortable in a position that is at least partially corrective for their curvature pattern. Precise instruction is necessary so patients are educated on how to change habits properly.

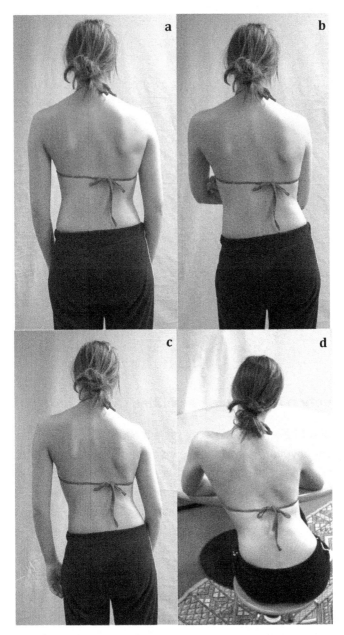

Fig. 7.11: (a) Patient with scoliosis pattern 3C, on the left uncorrected, on the right **(b)** with load on the left leg, and **(c)** carrying out the "shoulder tilt." When sitting **(d)** the patient should try to support the frontal translation movement with the shoulder tilt, although the patient opens the smaller lumbar counter-curve by crossing the right leg over.

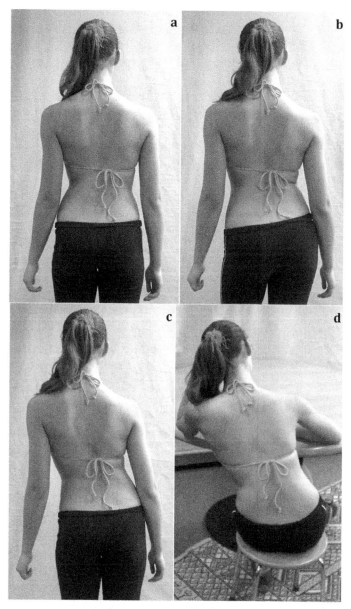

Fig. 7.12: (a) Patient with curvature pattern 3CH. In this case, the load is applied to the leg on the left side **(b)** particularly because there is no significant lumbar countercurve and focus can be on correcting the left-protruding hip to the right **(c).** When sitting, the right leg can be crossed over **(d).**

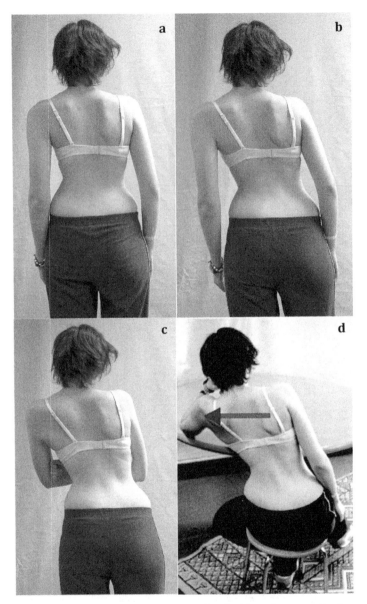

Fig. 7.13: (a) Patient with curvature pattern 4C with a double major curve. During everyday activities one must take care to introduce a translation movement to the left **(b)** which is supported by the shoulder girdle shift to the left. Here, it is important that the right pelvis not be raised, in order to open the lumbar curvature **(c).** When seated, the left leg is crossed to keep the right pelvis down **(d).**

There seems to be a mechanism according to which a mental engram is developed during the execution of exercises – a process which when carried out in inpatient conditions can be as much as five-and-one-half hours or more each day allowing the patient to experience the corrected posture. However, in some instances this engram seems to be switched off immediately once the exercise period is over, or even eliminated from the patient's awareness. This might be linked to the fact that the scoliosis is internalized as a deforming disease, with negativity, and may cause an individual to subconsciously reject everyday management (ADL). Consequently, it is crucial to integrate exercise and everyday activities. What is the correct relaxed sitting position? What is the correct lying position? How can one best lean against something while standing? These questions can only be answered via analysis of each individual case.

With radiological single curve patterns, the approach is simple. The patient must be instructed in postures that open up the major curvature in positions of rest. However, with double curve patterns, both major curvatures must be taken into account with resting positions, which is why a longer training period is necessary for this pattern of curvature. In Figures 7.11a-d, 7.12a-d, 7.13a-d, and 7.14a-d the possibilities for the appropriate patterns of curvature are demonstrated. The instruction concerning everyday rest positions must be considered separately from Lehnert-Schroth's thoroughly thought out correction program for the three-dimensional scoliosis treatment. It is not possible to take all functional equalization curvatures into consideration during one of these everyday rest positions. The main aim is to avoid 'hanging' in the major curvature in a way that encourages progression.

The following rules should be considered:

1. Radiologic single curvatures, including thoracic, thoracolumbar, or lumbar:

   a. When standing and sitting, leaning should be done principally to the concave side to open up this side.

   b. Lying should be on a soft bed on the concave side of the single curvature so that this can droop.

When lying in bed, the aim is not to regulate sleeping positions, but rather for the patient to become accustomed to a lying position that can be internalized over time and perhaps be adopted during sleep. This is difficult to accomplish, but worth striving for because even two hours spent reading in bed can have a negative effect when on the wrong side, and a positive effect when on the correct side (Fig. 7.15–7.17).

2. Radiologic double patterns of curvature:

   a. When standing and sitting, the patient should lean to the thoracic concave side; a sinking of the thoracic convex side pelvic half should also be achieved when sitting and standing by letting the thoracic concave side leg take on the burden.

   b. Lying should be done on a soft bed: for this, no general recommendations can be given since in the case of two opposing major curvatures, one curvature will always be encouraged when lying on soft bedding.

   One can, however, recommend that with radiologic double curve patterns, hard bedding be chosen since this will at least address the lower-lying curvature.

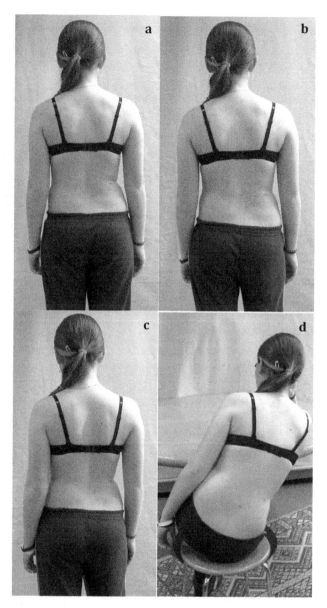

Fig. 7.14: (a) Patient with functional curvature pattern 4C with single curve lumbar scoliosis. In this case, during everyday activity, focus does not need to be on the smaller thoracic secondary curvature. The main visible feature is the hip protruding to the right, which can be centered with an appropriate loading on the left side while standing **(b and c)**. When sitting, the load should lie in the right lateral gluteal region, which automatically brings the pelvis to the left in the direction of correction, opposing gravity **(d)**.

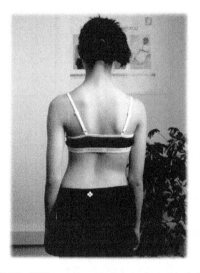
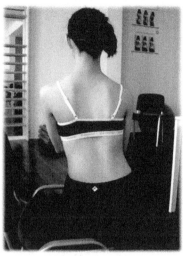

Fig. 7.15: Sitting on a stool in a lop-sided fashion. The patient (pattern 3CH, still very flexible) cannot lean to the right into the costal hump without slipping from the stool. Therefore, an automatic correction of the posture is carried out in the frontal plane without previous skills or previous practice.

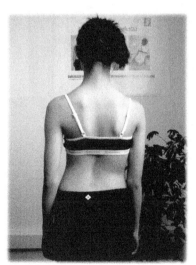
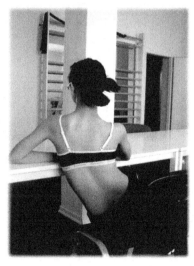

Fig. 7.16 "Wipe your neighbor away from the table!" The patient (pattern 3CH, still very flexible) can completely correct her curvature using this exercise from the *ADL* program. The right hip can move upwards. The patient therefore crosses her right leg (the leg on the costal hump side) over the left leg. For pattern 4C, the left leg (the leg on the costal cavity side) must be crossed over the right leg in order to prevent the right hip from moving upward. In doing so, a worsening of the lumbar countercurve can be prevented.

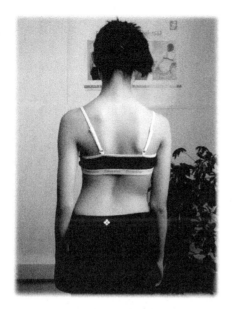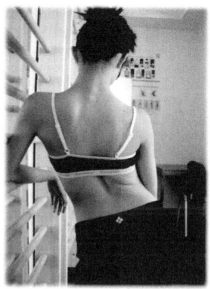

Fig. 7.17: Leaning to the thoracic concave side using the wooden bars. The patient (pattern 3CH, still very flexible) can completely correct her curvature using this exercise from the ADL program. She is making a correction in the sagittal plane that improves the thoracic flat-back (chin out).

7.3 The program 3D made easy

The program 3D made easy has been derived from everyday activities (ADLs). In principle, every exercise is initially learned in a standing position, but the everyday posture can be strengthened from a seated position as well. Two exercises form the basis: one exercise for the treatment of functional 3-curve scoliosis (thoracic scoliosis, 3CH, 3C, 3CTL) and one for the treatment of functional 4-curve scoliosis (double major, lumbar scoliosis, 4C, 4CL, 4CTL, and the pseudo functional 4-curve scoliosis 3CL).

These exercises are easy to learn (Weiss 2010) and ideally suited for mild curvatures, or in combination with the physio-logic® program. These exercises have been tested in a prospective and controlled fashion in 2006 and were judged relatively time-saving (Weiss, Hollaender and Klein 2006). One exercise (3D made easy), consists of four stages that always proceed in the same order:

- pelvic corrections in the frontal plane;
- spiral-form shoulder girdle correction (3D);
- selective breathing into the weak side, and
- maximal tensing of the trunk muscles in optimal correction.

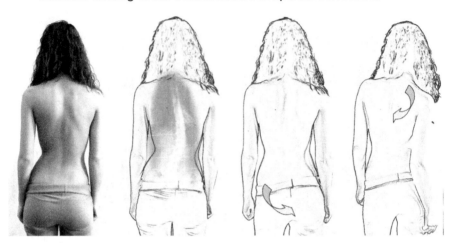

Fig. 7.18: 3D made easy for the treatment of curvatures of category 3C (with the exception of 3CL). On the *far left* we see the clinical image; *middle left* is the schematic diagram with x-ray; *middle right* is the pelvis correction with the shifting of the hip under the costal hump and on the *right* is the pectoral girdle correction with retroversion/adduction of the shoulder blade, which also automatically corrects the sagittal profile. Finally, the patient breathes into the thoracic concavity and the correction result is stabilized with the muscles.

7.3.1 3D made easy for the treatment of a curvature pattern of category 3C (with the exception of 3CL)

The 3D made easy program for treating 3C pattern curvatures is an exercise for the best possible three-dimensional correction of a functional 3-curve scoliosis (with the exception of 3CL). In Figure 7.18, this exercise is represented for pattern 3CTL – it is carried out in the same way for patterns 3CH and 3C. The treatment of functional 3-curve scoliosis takes place in a step-by-step fashion.

Initially, the hip is shifted under the costal hump by buckling the thoracic concave side leg (1).

Subsequently, the shoulder girdle correction takes place with retroversion/adduction of the shoulder blade of the thoracic convex side; the sagittal profile is also corrected through this process (2).

Through the opening up of the thoracic concave side, which has now been achieved, and through intentional guidance, the breath is directed into the concavity, correcting the ribs (that are rotated ventrally) in a dorsal direction (3).

At the end of the correction, the trunk musculature should be tensed completely during the breathing-out phase in order for the tension pattern to be better perceived (4).

7.3.2 3D made easy for the treatment of a curvature pattern of category 4C (including 3CL)

3D made easy for treating 4C pattern curvatures is an exercise for the best possible three-dimensional correction of a functional 4-curve scoliosis (including 3CL). In Figure 7.19 the exercise is represented for pattern 3CL – it is carried out in the same way for pattern 4C and, if necessary, for patterns 4CL and 4CTL. The treatment of functional 4-curve scoliosis takes place in a step-by-step fashion as well.

Initially, the hip is shifted under the lumbar bulge by buckling the thoracic convex side leg (1).

Subsequently, the shoulder girdle correction takes place with retroversion/adduction of the shoulder blade of the thoracic convex side; the sagittal profile is also corrected automatically by this process (2).

Through the opening up of the thoracic concave side and through intentional guidance the breath is directed into the concavity, correcting the ribs (that are rotated ventrally) in a dorsal direction (3).

At the end of the correction, the trunk musculature should be tensed in total during the breathing-out phase in order for the tension pattern to be better perceived (4).

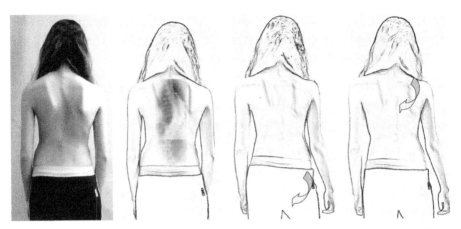

Fig. 7.19: 3D made easy for the treatment of curvatures of category 4C (including 3CL). On the *far left* we see the clinical image; *middle left* is the schematic diagram with x-ray; *middle right* is the pelvis correction with the shifting of the hip under the lumbar bulge and on the *right* the pectoral girdle correction with retroversion/adduction of the shoulder blade, which also automatically corrects the sagittal profile. Finally, the patient breathes into the thoracic concavity and the correction result is stabilized with the muscles.

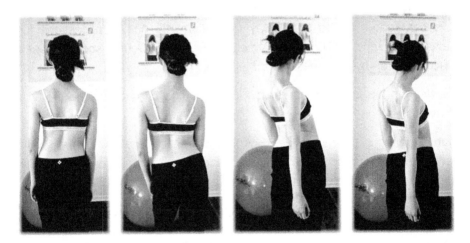

Fig. 7.20: 3D made easy for the treatment of curvatures of category 3C (with the exception of 3CL). On the *far left* we see the clinical image of a patient at rest; *middle left* is the pelvis correction with shifting of the hip under the costal hump; *middle right* is the pectoral girdle correction with retroversion/adduction of the shoulder blade, which also automatically results in a correction of the sagittal profile. Finally, the patient breathes into the thoracic concavity and the correction result is stabilized with the muscles (*right*).

Corrections are much harder to achieve with a functional 4-curve pattern of curvature than with a functional 3-curve pattern. The benefits of the compensated functional 4-curve patterns, however, are cosmetically less obvious and are less likely to increase after completion of growth (Asher and Burton 2006). The exercises from this program are effective and assist the patient when incorporating exercises from the Lehnert-Schroth program. These are also ideal "preliminary exercises" for the Schroth program in cases of more severe curvatures. In addition, the fundamental differences between functional 3 and 4-curves in the approach to exercises are demonstrated in the 3D made easy program. The sole difference is the positioning of the pelvis. In the frontal plane, the pelvis is shifted under the costal hump with a functional 3-curve scoliosis (Fig. 7.20) – i.e. to the parcel side – and is shifted to the weak side with a functional 4-curve scoliosis.

This principle is also maintained in the three-dimensional physiotherapy according to Lehnert-Schroth's method. It has been tailored according to the current state of scientific knowledge, which has made it possible to increase the 3D correction effect further. Hence, this treatment technique is termed "Power Schroth."

7.4 "Power Schroth" – the advanced development of three-dimensional scoliosis treatment according to Katharina Schroth's method

The original Schroth program consisted entirely of exercises for the treatment of functional 3-curve scoliosis. It was only in the 1970s that the functional 4-curve scoliosis was discovered by Lehnert-Schroth, along with the functional leg shortening that accompanies this curvature pattern. Scoliosis was thus classified accordingly, allowing for the most appropriate therapy based on the curve pattern. The Lehnert-Schroth classification (functional 3-curve scoliosis/functional 4-curve scoliosis) was also used by Chêneau in his construction of pattern-specific braces. As noted in the previous chapter, this classification remains in use today. However, the classifications that are widely used today are more precise, but are also more complex, and therefore, more difficult to understand.

In the previous edition of this book, Schroth's exercises for the various patterns of curvature were presented. However, three-dimensional scoliosis treatment according to Katharina Schroth's method is by no means a simple collection of exercises; it is more a principle of treatment. The multitude of exercises presented in Lehnert-Schroth's book was developed in order to provide patients with a certain amount of variation in their exercises during participation in a three to six month rehabilitation program. This historical meaning is often misunderstood today, which is precisely why a multitude of exercises often obscure the principles behind them.

In this chapter, we therefore focus on the principle of the exercises, rather than presenting a confusing multitude of different exercises for different patterns of curvature, particularly since these exercises are presented in the book, *Three-Dimensional Treatment* for *Scoliosis*, from Christa Lehnert-Schroth – a work of great historical significance (2007).

The exercises in the selection described by Lehnert-Schroth can always be used with functional 3-curve or functional 4-curve patterns. It has become standard practice for therapists to perform the majority of the exercises in a lying position while crouching near the patient in attempt to provide corrective assistance. However, this means that in this starting position an important "correction booster" is lacking, namely the use of automatic corrective positioning reflexes. It is precisely these positioning reflexes that are absolutely essential for constructing a corrected sense of posture, because it is only via asymmetric trunk muscle tension that the corrected posture can be perceived (Chapter 3). With the patient lying down, the therapist must work laboriously on the asymmetric correction tension, alongside many other elements of the exercises (props, intricacies of the exercise) that demand one's attention. However, in an upright position it happens automatically.

It has become typical to use many aids in the exercises (Fig. 7.21). Stools, rolling devices, cushions, elastic bands, and many other objects are used, even though they neglect to take the importance of everyday activities into account. The exercises have tended to become more acrobatic and about themselves, resulting in an exercise with no significant engram processed for application in everyday life. Therefore, nothing is applied which can contribute to the correction or relief of the distorted spine during daily activities. Of significant importance is a simplification of the exercises to focus the patient's attention on the sense of posture, and also to make the exercises more relevant to everyday activities. The goal is to influence the patient's everyday activities via beneficial movements and exercises, since with only twenty minutes per day of exercises, one cannot make a significant impression on the prognosis of scoliosis.

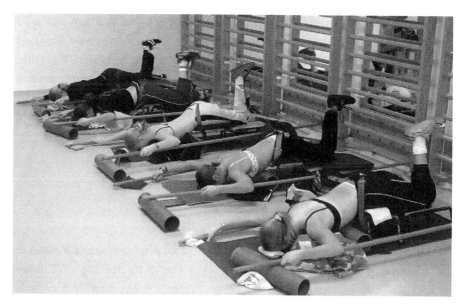

Fig. 7.21: It has become prevalent to carry out the majority of exercises in a horizontal position. Furthermore, it has become commonplace to employ more and more aids during the exercises. Stools, rolling devices, cushions, and elastic bands are used for the exercises, which only removes the patient further from everyday activities. This tendency is not a positive practice, particularly since flatback is actually worsened in this position.

Therefore, it is necessary to concentrate on only five important exercises in the program, along with simple tactile stimulation reminders which a practitioner can use effectively to help the patient facilitate the execution of the exercise. When utilizing these simple techniques, the patient need only recall the therapeutic reminders to be able to trigger the optimal attitude for the exercise automatically and without "wooden hip bars" [Hüftholz], or other aids which are not always readily available. Since these aids were not available at the beginning of the development of this method, it is justified in seeing this approach to the exercises as "Ur-Schroth" – as the original approach to the treatment, which was the starting point for the global expansion of the method.

Finally, the most recent insights regarding the extremity-induced synergism should be recognized: when both arms are brought into an elevated position, this leads to an anti-kyphotic synergy in the thoracic spine. If both arms are placed into retroversion (and if necessary, also into abduction), then a kyphosis-inducing synergy in the region of the thoracic spine is achieved. However, if the arm on the parcel side is brought into an elevated position and the arm on the weak side is brought into retroversion, then one achieves an anti-kyphosis-inducing effect on the parcel side and a kyphosis-inducing effect on the weak side that specifically and selectively counteracts the thoracic concave side flatback - generally desired with idiopathic scoliosis.

The position of the arms when using the new "Power Schroth" treatment is herewith clearly defined. A deviation is allowed with the rare kyphoscoliosis.

7.4.1 The muscle cylinder

The muscle cylinder can be carried out on the knees – as we described in the previous edition – on the side, or in a standing position. We have chosen the last of these positions here, since this is probably the most effective and, at the same time, the most pleasant starting position for the execution of this exercise, which, with an upright starting position, is highly laborious.

This exercise addresses the autochthonous back musculature unilaterally: in the lumbar region it addresses the intrinsically lumbar part that is characterized by an oblique orientation from the pelvis up to the transverse processes. As a result, a de-rotation of the lumbar concave side transverse processes (which are twisted in a ventral direction) occurs, while simultaneously erecting the lumbar curvature. In the thoracic spinal region, the autochthonous back musculature pulls in more of a longitudinal direction and is able to erect the thoracic convex side and simultaneously de-rotate. For this reason, the muscle cylinder is equally suited to triple and functional 4-curve curvatures (Fig. 7.22–7.23).

3B

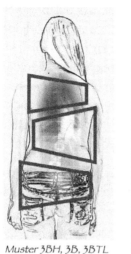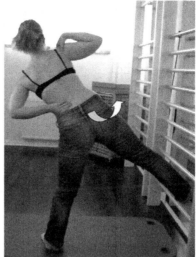

Muster 3BH, 3B, 3BTL

Fig. 7.22: Muscle cylinder being executed – functional 3-curve (German: 3B; 3-bogig) with pelvis position either straight or tilted under the parcel.

4B

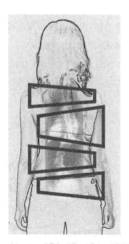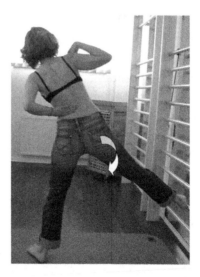

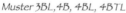

Muster 3BL, 4B, 4BL, 4BTL

Fig. 7.23: Muscle cylinder being executed – functional 4-curve (German: 4B; 4-bogig) with pelvis position either straight or tilted under to the weak side. The last-mentioned execution is, however, very difficult and is not possible with all patients. However, with a straight pelvis position, this exercise is ideal for both patterns.

173

Starting position

The leg on the thoracic convex side lies stretched out on its side, on a support of some kind (stool, wooden gymnastic bars). The upper body is lowered to the thoracic concave side, as an extension of this leg. The deflection of the thoracic convexity is led through the "shoulder counter-tension[1]" on the thoracic convex side. Simultaneously, the thoracic concavity can additionally be opened up via a concave side shoulder tension, obliquely, out of the concavity, and in the case of flatback, out of the inner rotation position of the thoracic concave-side arm.

The starting position is completed with a physiological sagittal positioning with tilted pelvis and ventralization of the costal arches (see also physiologic® program).

Active corrections

Prior to executing the standing muscle cylinder, a pre-correction of the deformity in the thoracic and lumbar region must be established. In the case of thoracic major curvatures, a clinical overcorrection of the curvature of the thoracic spine via an increase of the concave side shoulder tension should occur. With pronounced lumbar curvatures, the pelvis should be lowered on the thoracic convex side via a forefoot push with the thoracic convex side leg (to create the desired lordosis rather than the heel push used earlier), thereby opening up the lumbar curvature. However, the thoracic correction should not disappear in the process.

The rotational breathing technique

The Schroth rotational breathing technique enables further improvement of the corrections, as well as the approach to one's posture. The patient breathes in, selectively, into the thoracic concave side (weak side) in a

---

[1] "Shoulder counter-tension" and "shoulder tension" describe the efforts of the patient to push strongly outwards with the shoulders in the frontal plane. The shoulder counter-tension takes place on the thoracic convex side and is the cranial resistance against the costal hump correction in the frontal plane. In contrast, the shoulder tension helps to open up the thoracic concave side and thus leads the thoracic shift to the thoracic concave side.

lateral/dorsal direction and the ribs that are oriented ventrally are de-rotated dorsally; this correction is, if possible, increased with every inhalation. Skilled patients can selectively effect a correction of the thoracic concave side (weak side) or the lumbar concave side (weak spot), or both areas simultaneously.

Stabilization

After using the rotational breathing technique in the inhalation phase, in every subsequent exhalation the trunk musculature is tensed as much as possible with an optimal overall correction. In this way, depending on the condition of the patient, the inhalation correction from the rotational breathing and the tension during exhalation can be repeated many times. It is, however, required that the patient be able to keep up the fundamental correction.

7.4.2 The 50x exercise

Katharina Schroth's original 50x exercise is described in various ways in the literature. Initially, it was meant to be executed in a cross-legged position with corrections during inhalation with the task being to pull oneself upwards on the wooden wall bars during the exhalation phase. However, the cross-legged position leads to a kyphosis in the lumbar region and therefore contradicts current knowledge since the sagittal profile must also be taken into consideration during treatment. For this reason, one needs a higher sitting position. This can be achieved by sitting on an exercise ball or appropriate stool. This allows a slight lordotic positioning of the lumbar spine (Fig. 7.24–7.25).

Starting position

The patient sits on the exercise ball in a frontal position, in front of the wooden wall bars; the thighs are abducted and rotated outwards to create a stable starting position. The starting position is actually oriented towards the frame of the wooden wall bars on the thoracic convex side (parcel side), to allow for a lateral shift to the weak side.

3B

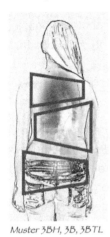

Muster 3BH, 3B, 3BTL

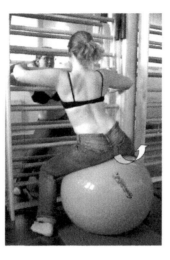

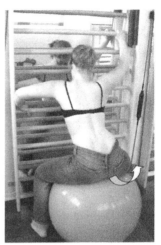

Fig. 7.24: 50x exercise being executed – functional 3-curve with pelvis position straight or tilted under to the parcel side. In the *middle*, the execution for an anti-kyphotic kyphoscoliosis; on the *right*, the execution for idiopathic scoliosis with thoracic flatback.

4B

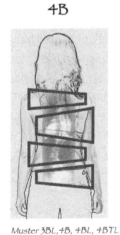

Muster 3BL,4B, 4BL, 4BTL

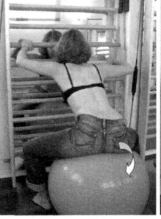

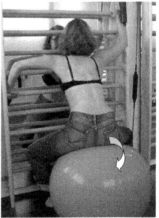

Fig. 7.25: 50x exercise being executed – functional 4-curve with pelvis position tilted under to the weak side. In the *middle*, the execution for an anti-kyphotic kyphoscoliosis; on the *right*, the execution for idiopathic scoliosis with thoracic flatback.

176

The hand on the parcel side grabs hold of a bar at eye level, one hand width medial of the frame; the hand on the weak side grabs hold of a bar at waist level, one hand width medial of the frame. Both elbows are bent so that the upper arms are oriented as parallel to the plane of the bars as possible in the frontal plane. Via the orientation of the starting position, around the frame, on the thoracic convex side (parcel side), the patient must perform an oblique pull to the thoracic concave side (weak side), thus opening up the weak side.

In the case of functional 3-curve scoliosis, the pelvis, on the weak side, is allowed to roll a little on the ball towards the thoracic convex side (parcel side); in the case of functional 3-curve scoliosis with structural lumbar countercurve, a neutral pelvic position is favored. In the case of functional 4-curve scoliosis, the pelvis remains horizontal on the ball and the half of the pelvis on the parcel side is lowered as much as possible.

Active corrections

Prior to executing the the 50x exercise, a pre-correction of the deformity in the thoracic and lumbar region must be established. In the case of thoracic major curvatures, a clinical overcorrection of the curvature of the thoracic spine via an increase of the concave side shoulder tension should occur. With pronounced lumbar curvatures, the pelvis should be lowered on the thoracic convex side, thereby opening up the lumbar curvature. However, the thoracic correction should not disappear in the process.

Rotational breathing

The rotational breathing technique enables further improvement of the corrections as well as the approach to one's posture. One breathes in, selectively, into the thoracic concave side (weak side) in a dorsal direction and the ribs that are oriented ventrally are de-rotated dorsally; this correction is, if possible, increased with every inhalation. Skilled patients can selectively effect a correction of the thoracic concave side (weak side) or the lumbar concave side (weak spot), or both areas simultaneously.

Stabilization

After using the rotational breathing technique in the inhalation phase, in every subsequent exhalation the trunk musculature is tensed as much as possible with an optimal overall correction. In this way, depending on the condition of the patient, the inhalation correction from the rotational breathing and the tension during exhalation can be repeated many times. It is, however, required that the patient be able to keep up the fundamental correction.

In addition, in the case of thoracic flatback, one of two things can be performed: either the arm on the weak side is pressed inwards against the bar during the exhalation phase, or the elbow on the weak side is held firmly against resistance provided by the therapist (later also virtual resistance).

7.4.3 The door handle exercise

Just like the 50x exercise, the original exercise is described with a deep sitting starting position. However, the cross-legged position leads to a kyphosis in the lumbar region and therefore contradicts current knowledge, which says that the sagittal profile must also be taken into consideration during treatment. For this reason, one needs a somewhat higher sitting position, e.g. by sitting on an exercise ball. In addition, this allows a slight lordotic positioning of the lumbar spine (Fig. 7.26–7.27). In the original version of the exercise, the patient was meant to pull upwards using the arm on the weak side – which is rotated outward – but this clearly favors flatback. For this reason, this exercise is still used in its original version with kyphoscoliosis.

Starting position

The patient sits on the exercise ball in front of the wooden wall bars; the thighs are abducted and rotated outwards in order to create a stable starting position – the thoracic concave side is turned laterally toward the wooden wall bars.

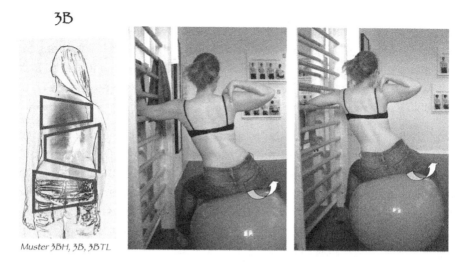

Muster 3BH, 3B, 3BTL

Fig. 7.26: The new door handle exercise being executed – functional 3-curve with pelvis position straight or tilted under the parcel. In the *middle*, the execution for a kyphoscoliosis; on the *right*, the execution for idiopathic scoliosis with thoracic flatback.

4B

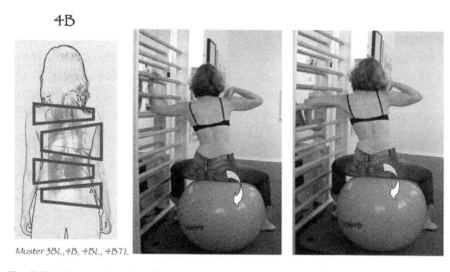

Muster 3BL, 4B, 4BL, 4BTL

Fig. 7.27: The new door handle exercise being executed – functional 4-curve with pelvis position tilted under the weak side. This is achieved through caudalization of the thoracic convex side half of the pelvis. In the *middle*, the execution for a kyphoscoliosis; on the *right*, the execution for idiopathic scoliosis with thoracic flatback.

The hand on the parcel side grabs hold of the shoulder on the parcel side for shoulder counter-traction; the upper arm is positioned to act as an extension of the shoulder girdle plane; the hand on the weak side grabs the bar at waist level through the gap between the bars at shoulder level. Both elbows are bent so that the upper arms are oriented as vertically as possible to the wall bar in the frontal plane.

Due to the starting position being at a distance from the wall bars, an oblique tension is applied to the thoracic concave side (weak side) and thus, the weak side is opened up. In the case of functional 3-curve scoliosis, the pelvis on the weak side is lowered slightly on the exercise ball toward the wall bars; in the case of functional 3-curve scoliosis with structural lumbar countercurve, a neutral pelvic position is favored. In the case of functional 4-curve scoliosis, the pelvis remains horizontal on the ball and the half of the pelvis on the parcel side is lowered as much as possible.

Active corrections

Prior to executing the door handle exercise, a pre-correction of the deformity in the thoracic and lumbar region must be established. In the case of thoracic major curvatures, a clinical overcorrection of the curvature of the thoracic spine via an increase of the concave side shoulder tension should occur. With pronounced lumbar curvatures, the pelvis should be lowered on the thoracic convex side. However, the thoracic correction should not disappear in the process.

Schroth rotational breathing

The rotational breathing technique enables further improvement of the corrections as well as the approach to the patient's posture. One breathes in, selectively, into the thoracic concave side (weak side) in a dorsal direction and the ribs that are oriented ventrally are de-rotated dorsally; this correction is, if possible, increased with every inhalation. Skilled patients can selectively effect a correction of the thoracic concave side (weak side) or the lumbar concave side (weak spot), or both areas simultaneously.

Stabilization

After using the rotational breathing technique in the inhalation phase, in every subsequent exhalation the trunk musculature is tensed as much as possible with an optimal overall correction. In this way, depending on the condition of the patient, the inhalation correction from the rotational breathing and the tension during exhalation can be repeated many times. The patient is required to keep up the fundamental correction.

In addition, in the case of thoracic flatback, the exercise can be performed one of two ways: either the arm on the weak side is pressed inward against the bar during the exhalation phase, or with the patient grasping the wall with his/her hand, on the weak side, squeezing firmly while maintaining a stationary position and pulling back with the hand during the exhalation phase.

7.4.4 The frog at the pond

The muscle cylinder can be carried out at home without any aids; the 50x exercise and the new door handle exercise can be carried out using a doorframe or chair. However, achieving the motivation to carry out these exercises without the wooden wall bars is not easy. Therefore, a new exercise has been developed which is designed to have the same effect, and can be performed at home without any aids. This new "Power Schroth" exercise, called the frog at the pond, satisfies these demands (Fig. 7.28–7.29).

Starting position

The patient sits back on their heels with their legs folded under them, on soft padding with the knees hip-width apart. The hand on the weak side is positioned next to the knee on the weak side with a straightened elbow with the same spacing as the distance between the knees. The hand on the parcel side grabs hold of the same shoulder, on the parcel side, to provide shoulder counter-tension, with the upper-arm positioned so as to be an extension of the shoulder girdle plane.

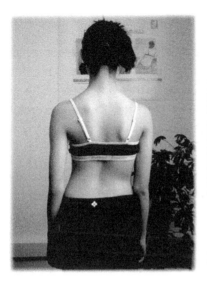
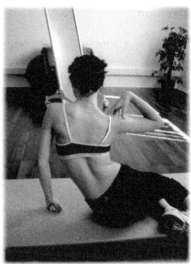

Fig. 7.28: The "frog at the pond" exercise being executed – functional 3-curve with pelvis position tilted under the parcel (sitting, with legs folded back, heels folded back next to the body). The patient has a thoracic curvature of 43°, however, since she is only twelve years old, she is still very flexible.

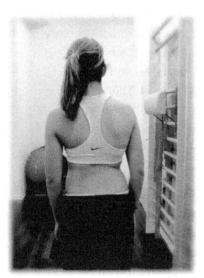
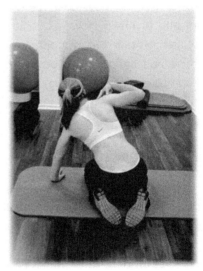

Fig. 7.29: The "frog at the pond" exercise being executed – functional 4-curve with horizontally stabilized pelvis position (legs folded under the buttocks, sitting on the heels). In this way, the right half of the pelvis is prevented from coming free, which protects the lumbar correction. The nearly fifteen-year-old patient is classified as 3CL with a stiff thoracic curvature with a 50° Cobb angle.

Active corrections

Prior to executing the frog at the pond, a pre-correction of the deformity in the thoracic and lumbar region must be established. The goal is to achieve a reduction of the flatback by a retroversion of the arm on the weak side against resistance from the floor (kyphosis-inducing synergy).

In the case of pronounced lumbar curvatures (functional 4-curve), the pelvis should be lowered on the thoracic convex side, which opens up the lumbar curvature. This is encouraged through the starting position, in which the pelvis is fixed parallel to the floor (Fig. 7.29). However, in doing so, the shift movement to the thoracic concave side becomes more difficult. With functional 3-curve scoliosis, one can try to position the pelvis on the weak side next to the lower leg, which will open up a drawn out thoracic curvature (Fig. 7.28).

Schroth rotational breathing

The rotational breathing technique enables further improvement of the corrections as well as the approach to the patient's posture. One breathes in, selectively, into the thoracic concave side (weak side) in a dorsal direction and the ribs that are oriented ventrally are de-rotated dorsally; this correction is, if possible, increased with every inhalation. Skilled patients can selectively effect a correction of the thoracic concave side (weak side) or the lumbar concave side (weak spot), or both areas simultaneously.

Stabilization

After using the rotational breathing technique in the inhalation phase, in every subsequent exhalation the trunk musculature is tensed as much as possible with an optimal overall correction. In this way, depending on the condition of the patient, the inhalation correction from the rotational breathing and the tension during exhalation can be repeated many times. However, the patient is required to keep up the fundamental correction.

Depending on the patient, during the exhalation phase the arm on the weak side can be tensed against resistance from the floor in a ventral lateral or ventral medial direction; however, with thoracic flatback the resistance should be pushed against in a dorsal direction.

7.4.5 Raising the pelvis

Raising the pelvis is an original exercise derived from Christa Lehnert-Schroth's collection. It is actually more energy-draining than specific. However, it is presented here to satisfy patients who desire additional intensity.

This exercise can be tailored specifically for triple or functional 4-curve scoliosis, if the patient's strength is sufficient. The fundamental principle of Schroth exercise execution, the inhalation with correction of the concavities and the trunk muscle tension during exhalation phase, are all employed.

It is quite an achievement to use the exercise nonspecifically for the correction of a thoracic curvature. With functional 3-curve execution, the top leg is bent slightly, and the pelvis is lifted slightly through the abduction of the lower leg. In the functional 4-curve execution, the bottom leg is bent and the upper leg is straightened in order to open up the lumbar curvature; the pelvis is raised through the adduction of the upper lying leg (Fig. 7.30-7.31).

Starting position

The patient lies on their side on soft padding, propped up on their elbow on the weak side. The hand on the weak side is resting on the floor as far as possible in a caudal direction in order to achieve an inward twisting of the arm on the weak side (kyphotic synergy against the concave side flatback). The hand on the parcel side grabs hold of the shoulder on the parcel side to create shoulder counter-tension, with the upper arm positioned so as to be an extension of the shoulder girdle plane.

Active corrections

Prior to executing the raising the pelvis exercise, a pre-correction of the deformity in the thoracic and lumbar region must be established, as explained above.

With the functional 3-curve execution, the top leg is slightly bent, the bottom leg is straightened, with the pelvis raised during the exhalation phase through the abduction of the lower leg. With the functional 4-curve execution, the bottom leg is bent and the top leg is straightened to open up the lumbar curvature. The pelvis is then raised during the exhalation phase through an adduction of the top leg with the help of an abduction of the lower leg (without the knee making contact with the floor).

3B

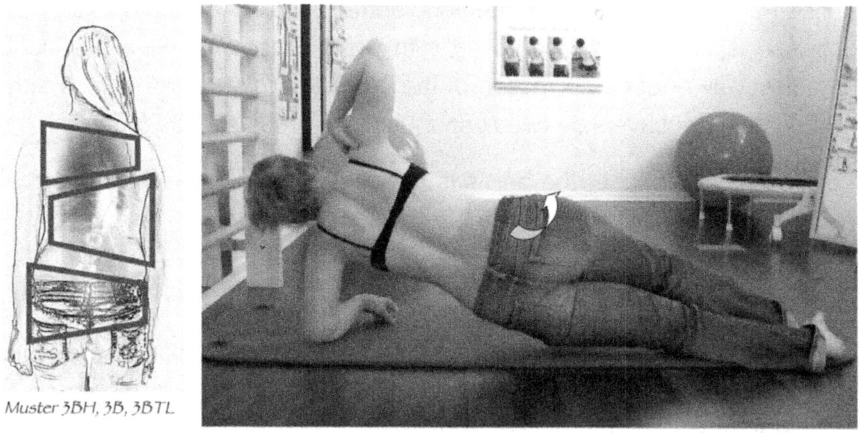

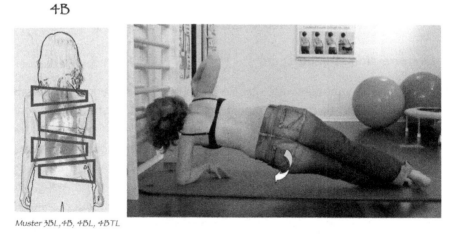

Muster 3BH, 3B, 3BTL

Fig. 7.30: Raising the pelvis exercise being executed – functional 3-curve. With the execution of this exercise, the leg lying on top is slightly bent and the pelvis is lifted over the abduction of the leg lying underneath.

4B

Muster 3BL, 4B, 4BL, 4BTL

Fig. 7.31: Raising the pelvis exercise being executed – functional 4-curve. With the execution of this exercise, the leg lying on the bottom is slightly bent and the pelvis is lifted over the adduction of the leg lying above. In doing so, the lumbar curvature opens up (see text).

Schroth rotational breathing

The rotational breathing technique enables further improvement of the corrections as well as the approach to the patient's posture. One breathes in, selectively, into the thoracic concave side (weak side) in a dorsal direction and the ribs that are oriented ventrally are de-rotated dorsally; this correction is, if possible, increased with every inhalation. Skilled patients can selectively effect a correction of the thoracic concave side (weak side) or the lumbar concave side (weak spot), or both areas simultaneously.

In the exhalation phase, the pelvis is raised and maintained for as long as possible for additional phases of the rotational breathing.

Stabilization

After using the rotational breathing technique in the inhalation phase, in every subsequent exhalation the trunk musculature is tensed as much as possible with an optimal overall correction. If possible, a reduction of the flatback is achieved through retroversion of the arm on the weak side against resistance from the floor (kyphosis-inducing synergy). Depending on the condition of the patient, the inhalation correction from the rotational breathing and the tension during exhalation can be repeated many times. However, the patient is required to keep up the fundamental correction.

7.4.6 Correction strengtheners

Correction strengtheners are tactile stimuli or resistances that are specifically applied by qualified practitioners. A correction strengthener can be, for example, the tactile stimulation of the weak side, if necessary, the weak point as well, in order to guide inhaled air into the hollow trunk area. Bridging stimuli are applied making it easier for the patient to intuitively comprehend the opening character of the corrective movement. Along with tactile stimuli, which are intended to promote the expansion of the concave trunk areas, there are also resistances against the corrective movement from the shoulder and pelvic girdle. These resistances are applied in the exhalation phase after rotational breathing has been executed.

Correction strengthener at the elbow on the weak side

During the 50x exercise, in the exhalation phase and with optimal alignment of the shoulder girdle with the upper arms, positioned in one line, a resistance is applied at the elbow on the weak side against the shoulder girdle shift to the thoracic concave side. This correction strengthener leads directly to increased tension of the thoracic convex side autochthonous back musculature. Practitioners must be careful not to apply or remove the resistances too abruptly and that the resistance is not so strong that the desired correction is lost.

Correction strengthener at the shoulder blade on the parcel side

For correction of thoracic curvatures, the shoulder blade on the parcel side plays a key role. Through resistance against the adduction/retroversion movement of the shoulder blade from the practitioner's thumb, the complex correction movement of the shoulder girdle is learned easily. Additionally, a feeling for posture and correction for everyday corrections with this pattern of curvature can be acquired quickly.

Initially, the thumb serves as a reference point for the shoulder blade. The adduction/retroversion movement is carried out as far as possible. With larger curvatures, initially this may seem insufficient; however, it's important to note that these curvatures can be very rigid. On the other hand, mild curvatures may be overcorrected using this maneuver and sometimes even without any additional corrections.

After the end-range position of the shoulder blade correction, the practitioner applies maximum resistance with their thumb allowing the patient to experience the tension/activation pattern necessary for the correction, and instructs the patient how to incorporate this maneuver into everyday activities.

This correction aid is used as a point of reference for facilitating the exercises from the 3D made easy program during the instruction phase. With the patterns 4C and 3CL, a counter-shift from the shoulder and pelvic girdle is desired. To facilitate this correction maneuver with these patterns, the focus is on the adduction correction of the shoulder blade to decrease the retroversion component.

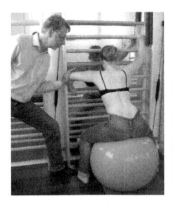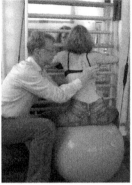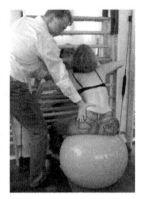

Fig. 7.32: Representation of the three most important correction boosters. Even after a brief period of learning, an engram for the correction value evolves and one only needs to remind the patient once that the appropriate resistances have been set and a clear increase in correction will be observed. This effect is called the "virtual therapist." On the *left*, the correction booster at the elbow joint on the weak side for the correction of thoracic curvatures. In the *middle*, the correction booster at the shoulder blade of the parcel side for the correction of thoracic curvatures. On the *right*, the correction booster at the iliac crest on the weak side for the correction of lumbar curvature.

Correction strengthener at the iliac crest on the weak side

For correction of a lumbar curvature, the dorsal iliac crest on the weak side plays a key role. Through resistance applied cranially of the spina iliaca posterior superior on the weak side against the dorsal positioning and the "cranialization" of this half of the pelvis by the practitioner's hand, the complex correction movement of the pelvic girdle can be learned easily. Additionally, a feeling for posture and correction for everyday corrections with functional 4-curve patterns of curvature can be acquired quickly.

We want to achieve a static overcorrection of the prominent pelvis, a "relordosation" and a simultaneous de-rotation of the lumbar bulge. The correction isn't always easy to achieve using this grasp; sometimes many post-corrections are necessary, perhaps because the pelvic position is less clearly determined in a person's posture engram.

The three most important correction strengtheners can be seen in Figure 7.32.

7.4.7 Peculiarities of functional 4-curve correction mechanisms

According to the clinical findings, with a functional 4-curve pattern, the hip on the parcel side protrudes. Logically, according to the original correction principles, this hip should be shifted medially. This is also possible with the simple functional 4-curve patterns 4CL and 4CTL, particularly since these patterns will present with a prominent hip as the major cosmetic feature. Interference of the pelvis corrections with the thoracic countercurve is minimal and, in fact, insignificant.

With patterns 4C and 3CL, we are concerned with a double curvature and both elements must be corrected. If one curvature is corrected too much, then the other curvature will be increased. Due to this challenge, some practitioners give in and accept a style of exercise that is more compensatory in nature and therefore, less effective. However, for this pattern of curvature, new and far more effective correction principles have been developed thanks to corrections occurring during Chêneau-brace treatment, as documented radiologically.

In the past, during brace treatment of pattern 4C, focus was only on recompensating the shoulder and pelvic girdle, and a very respectable and compensated clinical pattern of correction resulted. The cranial flank of the thoracic curvature and the caudal flank of the lumbar curvature became well erected, but tilted positioning of the neutral vertebra was always observed in the transition zone between the two curvatures, resulting in a Cobb angle that was still too large.

The only solution in this case is a trunk shift to the weak side with a simultaneous caudal positioning of the parcel side hip in order to open up the lumbar curve (Fig. 7.33). Relatively speaking, the parcel side hip still protrudes here, but the corrections that are achieved are excellent for this curve pattern.

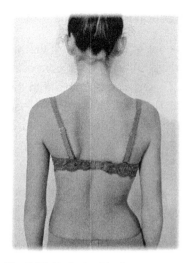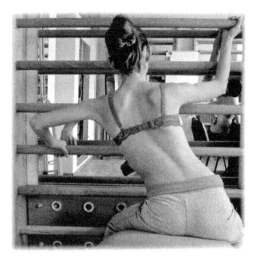

Fig. 7.33: Patient with the curvature pattern 4C, on the left in neutral position and on the right in the 50x exercise from the "New Power Schroth" program. One sees that it was possible to mirror not only the thoracic curvature, but also the lumbar major curvature in the exercise. Through the strong 'shift' to the thoracic concave side, the patient appears 'askew' in the exercise. (With kind permission of Maksym Borysov, bma-ukrniip@mail.ru, Kharkov, The Ukraine.)

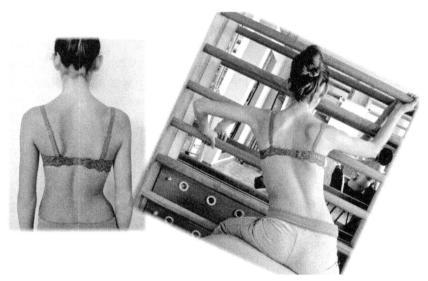

Fig. 7.34: If you turn the image of the patient (from Fig. 7.33) in the 50x exercise on its side, the scale of the correction achieved becomes clearly visible. Both curvatures are clinically over-corrected. (With kind permission of Maksym Borysov, bma-ukrniip@mail.ru, Kharkov, The Ukraine.)

Therefore, with both curve patterns, the maximum possible shift to the weak side must be attempted. However, one exception when considering treatment of triple and functional 4-curve scoliosis is the position of the pelvis. With functional 3-curve scoliosis, the pelvis can be tilted cranially on the parcel side. With functional 4-curve scoliosis (4C, 3CL, and with holistic treatment of the patterns 4CL and 4CTL including the thoracic correction in the early phase during the major growth spurt), the pelvis must be oriented caudally on the parcel side in order to open up the lumbar curvature. This is seen clearly when the exercise image in Figure 7.33 is tipped horizontally (Fig. 7.34). Further examples of exercises for functional 3- and functional 4-curve scoliosis can be seen in Figures 7.35–7.40.

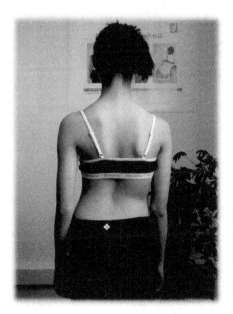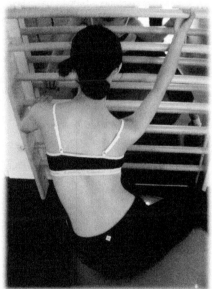

Fig. 7.35: A 12-year-old patient with a thoracic curvature of 43° Cobb angle; on the left, in a position of rest and on the right executing the 50x exercise – functional 3-curve. With this curvature pattern, the hip should be brought under the costal hump during the exercise. Since the patient is still young, the curvature is still relatively flexible and can thus be corrected well using this exercise.

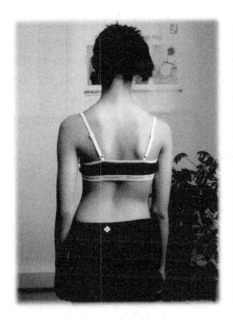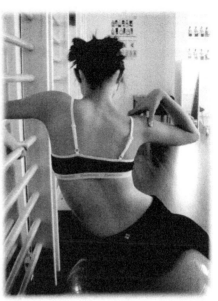

Fig. 7.36: A patient executing the door handle exercise.

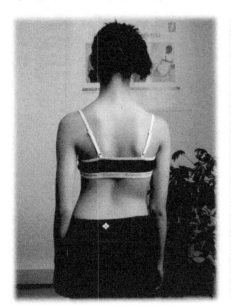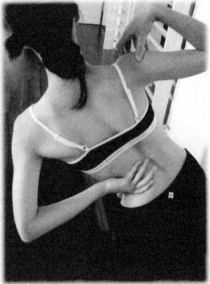

Fig. 7.37: A patient executing the muscle cylinder exercise. A correction of the sagittal profile is evident.

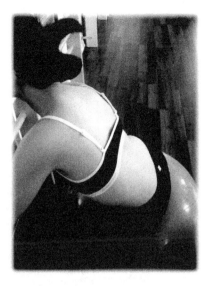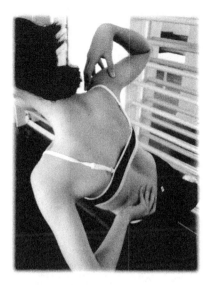

Fig. 7.38: A patient during exercises from the "New Power Schroth" program. In these images a good correction of the sagittal profile with a re-lordosis in the lumbar region and a re-kyphosis in the thoracic region is evident.

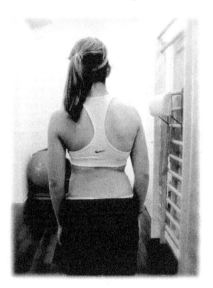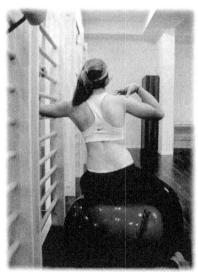

Fig. 7.39: This patient has a stiff thoracic curvature of 53°, pattern 3CL, initially treated as functional 4-curve. During the door handle exercise only a small recompensation to the left, thoracic concave side, is initially possible. The thigh on the thoracic convex side (parcel side) is lowered laterally to the caudal fixture of the pelvis and the foot is pushed in a dorsal direction and thus pushes the right, pushed-back half of the pelvis forward.

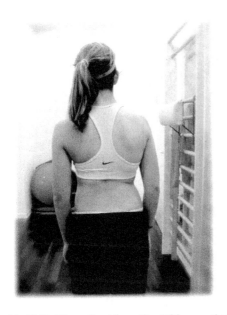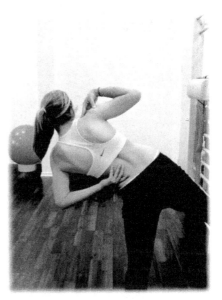

Fig. 7.40: The patient from Fig. 7.39 executing the muscle cylinder exercise. One can see an excellent correction of the trunk, although the position of the cervical spine is not yet optimal. Using an optimally practiced trunk position, this will eventually be improved. Ideally, the head position should be in line with the cervical spine which should should align with the thoracic and lumbar spine. After proper execution of the trunk corrections now head alignment can be improved further.

7.5 Walking rehabilitation

It is important to address walking, one of the most common everyday activities. The catwalk has been described previously. So, our focus will turn to education for walking rehabilitation.

As a basic symmetric pattern for correcting scoliosis in the sagittal plane, the catwalk can be expanded through asymmetric movements for 3D correction. 3D made easy is the basis for 3D correction while walking. As a result we have now elevated 3D correction to a higher statomotoric/ psychomotor level.

When executed optimally, rhythmically, and in a relaxed fashion, the catwalk can be used for locomotion, symmetrically, in various ways to facilitate 3D correction:

1. With patterns 3C, 3CH, and 3CTL, through an increase of the shoulder girdle rotation into the correction in accordance with the shoulder blade pattern described in the previous section: during the load-bearing phase of the leg on the parcel side, the patient shifts their shoulder girdle rhythmically from the parcel side to the weak side and simultaneously directs the parcel side shoulder blade in a caudal and medial direction.

2. With patterns 4CL and 4CTL, through an increase in the lateral pelvic tilt to the weak side: during the load-bearing phase of the leg on the weak side, the patient shifts – or oscillates – their shoulder girdle rhythmically, also to the weak side.

3. With patterns 4C and 3CL, through an increase in the lateral shift from the shoulder and pelvic girdles against each other (Fig. 7.41): during the load-bearing phase of the leg on the parcel side, the patient shifts their shoulder girdle to the weak side. The correction maneuvers described are to be rhythmically accentuated, increased and exaggerated, in accordance with the sequence of the steps. After, a correction that was conspicuous during exercise can then be downgraded in everyday situations. The best way to instruct the patient in 3D walking is on a treadmill; however, it is possible to teach this technique in a span of approximately thirty feet, but this requires slightly more effort on the part of the practitioner.

7.6 Short-term rehabilitation

There is now a record of short-term outpatient rehabilitation with children and adolescents. Training courses concerning posture can be carried out effectively in a matter of days. Patients learn how they can avoid everyday behaviors that promote their curvatures in scoliosis-specific back schools. In contrast, there is a lack of scientific results for the extended inpatient rehabilitation the way it is currently executed (Yilmaz and Kozikoglu 2010), meaning that improvements in the functional abilities of scoliosis patients has not been proven after the current available inpatient program.

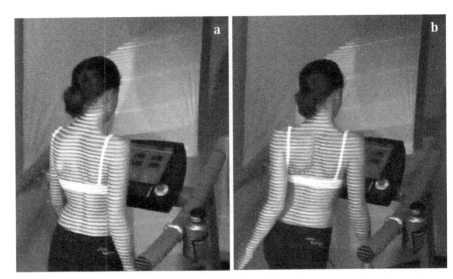

Fig. 7.41: Correction on the treadmill using simultaneous 3D analysis with the Formetric®
walking analysis. The patient has a left thoracic curvature of the 4C pattern **(a)** and, during
the load-bearing phase on the leg on the parcel side shifts her pectoral girdle
correspondingly in a rhythmic fashion over to the weak side, e.g. in this case to the right **(b)**.

When the patient training is carried out in a standardized way, quality of
results is consistent and reproducible objectives are attainable. Moreover,
the target for scoliosis treatment is clearly defined in Schroth Best Practice
methodology: it is for the development of a sense of posture and movement
that allows the patient to avoid behavior that encourages an increased
curvature. Therefore, focus shifts from the execution of a multitude of
exercises, with instantaneous correction, to a methodology promoting
objectives which include a sustainable educational result.

The group dynamic during inpatient rehabilitation may undoubtedly have a
positive effect on patients' motivation. Patients are visibly happy to meet
others experiencing similar circumstances. However, this social bonus is
more about a shared experience rather than the individual attainment of
specific abilities and skills. According to inpatient experiences, this means
that for camaraderie, inpatient rehabilitation is highly valued, but, over time
it is questionable that the educational objectives are able to be summoned
upon demand, in the long-term. This is likely due to the "schooling" concept
that is currently used in inpatient rehabilitation and its fixed teacher-pupil
setting which may simply lead to short-term memorization. Certainly, the

most motivated patients do learn from this didactic approach and are able to retain the concepts on a long-term basis, but others may experience difficulty. Furthermore, the first treatment week of inpatient rehabilitation consists of extensive theoretical content (anatomy, physiology etc.) rather than practical executions. This has little to do with improving the motivation necessary to help most patients accomplish their goals. In contrast, short-term outpatient rehabilitation has been modified, so the patient begins to learn exercise movements almost immediately. In the newest teaching approach, the didactic concepts have been abandoned and replaced with self-discovery, or experiential learning. The foremost reason for this is that when patients are taught to discover the needed concepts on their own, and develop their own sense of body awareness, they are more likely to retain those concepts over the long-term (Weiss 2012).

In the U.S., Moramarco's scoliosis-specific back school follows Schroth Best Practice, and patient instruction is often on a one-to-one basis. Some patients prefer the individual attention, time-efficiency, and scheduling flexibility. With individual instruction, what the patient lacks in companionship, they gain in depth and breadth of knowledge for their specific curve pattern and individualized activities. Peer support via referrals is provided for those individuals and families wanting to connect with other patients with similar circumstances.

Obviously, pros and cons exist for group versus individual instruction – from the patient's perspective, and from the practitioner's. Either way, when using Schroth Best Practice, the most important component of a successful outpatient rehabilitation approach is accomplished: experiential learning and the acquisition of the needed concepts to manage one's scoliosis over the long-term.

In fact, this is an additional benefit of short-term outpatient therapy – it allows for either group or individualized training and offers each patient the option for that flexibility based on learning style. The individual practitioner can decide which method suits his/her style and which method suits each particular patient best. Whichever approach is utilized, the patient can be sure that experiential learning and self-discovery will be an integral part of their short-term rehabilitation program and that the foundational concepts of focus will be:

- standardized learning content (for high process quality);
- the most modern pedagogical approaches;
- modern evidence-based rehabilitation methods (with established results).

The structure of the short rehabilitation program is outlined in the following section. Specific content can only be learned in the context of the practitioner training course.

Prior to starting the rehabilitation program, the physician must examine the patient, review x-rays and educate the patient on their scoliosis. It is helpful for the patient to understand their unique three-dimensional deformity prior to beginning the rehabilitation program. As part of the examination, scoliometer measurement, lung capacity and chest expansion should be assessed. These measurements are simple to perform and allow for progress monitoring without radiation.

Short scoliosis rehabilitation program

Day 1

Module 1: Meet-and-greet session, physio-logic® (standing, sitting, walking, catwalk);

Module 2: Self-discovery (experiential) learning: recognition of patterns of curvature;

Module 3: (a) physio-logic®, (b) Verification of patterns of curvature, (c) ADL (standing, sitting, and walking).

Day 2

Module 4: a, b, c, and (d) 3D made easy;

Module 5: Self-sufficient exercise practice (Objective: improved execution of exercises);

Module 6: Self-sufficient exercise practice (Objective: improved execution of exercises) a, b, c, d, and (e) Schroth exercise (50x exercise on ball and door handle exercise). 3D corrections are added and built into the catwalk walking training (a).

Day 3

Module 7: a, b, c, d, e, and (f) Muscle cylinder, the frog at the pond;

Module 8: Complete program with all exercises (self-sufficient improved execution of exercises);

Module 9: Practical test of the entire program (60 min.), optional written test (30 min.).

The individual modules last 90 – 120 min. The sequence of the contents must be adhered to for unified quality and results.

The short rehabilitation program (Weiss 2010, Borysov and Borysov 2012, Pugacheva 2012, Lee 2014) is not only geared toward treatment of children and adolescents, but also for adults who want to learn an effective scoliosis management program. Patients with severe secondary functional impairments (vital capacity, chronic pains) should seek individualized outpatient instruction by an experienced practitioner or look to inpatient treatment.

7.7 Physiotherapeutic treatment of scoliosis for children

The findings-specific exercises in the Schroth Best Practice program can be used in a routine fashion with most children. The exercises aim to develop postural awareness and are achieved through treatment protocols which show the patient how to integrate this awareness and new-found knowledge into everyday activities. The goal of scoliosis management is teaching the patient to avoid everyday behaviors which may encourage progression. It is a psychomotor conditioning process that always requires the active collaboration and concentration of the patient, especially initially. Some children under age ten lack necessary cognitive skills and are unable to engage in the active collaborative work to the extent required. Early in the learning process, significant effort is required by the patient since the goal is to find ways to influence the spinal curvature utilizing purely reflex mechanisms. Not all young children have the ability to sustain the necessary effort, so in this case we defer to PEP – described below (Weiss 1993).

Considering the knowledge that favorable posture reactions can be triggered through Feldenkrais exercises (awareness through movement) or the Vojta principles, corrective posture reactions were examined to determine to what extent those reactions can be encouraged in scoliosis patients through intensive facilitation. After investigating and understanding the principles behind these techniques, it became clear that through the starting positions for reflex crawling and reflex turning, the corrective route can sometimes become blocked. The Vojta grip technique was performed in a relaxed belly position allowing a certain corrective movement to be achieved by reflex. So, we had to consider that the human body instinctively tries to remove itself from external pressure as a type of fleeing reflex, and when it is impossible to flee, the body will instinctively put up resistance to this pressure. As a result, the following treatment technique has been developed and called periphery-evoking postural reaction (PEP).

7.7.1 Fundamental principles of the PEP exercises

The standard way of proceeding, as described below, is that a pressure is built up in the direction of the apical vertebra with both hands placed on the concave side. This pressure is held against the ribcage's breathing expansion for ten to twenty breaths. A flat contact between the hands and the concave side of the trunk deformity is necessary. This pressure is applied in the direction of the spinal distortion.

After ten to twenty breaths, the pressure is slowly released allowing the body to feel the region under pressure being released. In this instance, not only do the automatically correcting position reflexes activate themselves, but the previously pressed and pressurized region of the body triggers body awareness. Exercises, which include the shoulder and pelvic girdle are also possible. These exercises are used according to the pattern of curvature. With a lumbar curvature, the pelvic girdle can be integrated into the exercise; with a thoracic curvature, the shoulder girdle can also be integrated. In a slightly altered form, these exercises can also be integrated into the Schroth exercises to manifest the feeling of posture, and also to improve the breathing direction of the patient while performing the exercises.

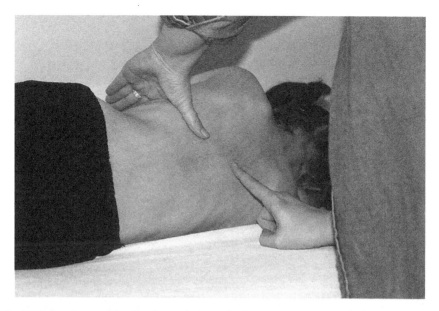

Fig. 7.42: Starting position for the treatment of a thoracic curvature with the PEP program in a lateral position on the costal hump side. The thoracic concave side is facing the therapist. The index finger is pointing to the thoracic apical vertebral region.

7.7.2 Description of exercises

The PEP program for the thoracic curvature

When performing PEP thoracic exercise (1), the patient lies on the thoracic convex side (Fig. 7.42). The practitioner fits the closed fingers of both hands up to the metacarpus bone to the contours of the body on the concave side of the trunk. The contact surfaces of the two hands are initially positioned parallel to the skin with a distance of one or two finger-widths between them (Fig. 7.43a). After, a pressure is applied into the concavities and the hands are brought together under increasing pressure. The pressure is shifted to the radial side of the hands (Fig. 7.43b). The pressure is held for twenty breaths and slowly reduced again with the inhalation phase; then, the hands slide away from each other.

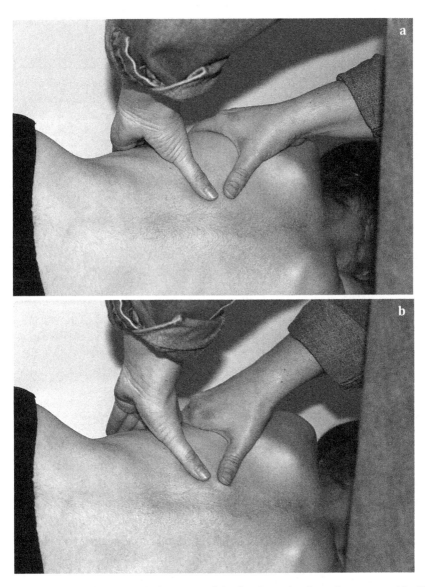

Fig. 7.43: (a) Two-dimensional alignment of the hands to the thoracic concave side. **(b)** There should be a small gap between the hands so that they can be brought together with increasing pressure. The pressure is transferred on the radial side of the hands and thus increased in the region of the curvature's apex. This pressure is held for twenty breaths and then slowly reduced with the inhalation phase (PEP exercise 1 thoracic).

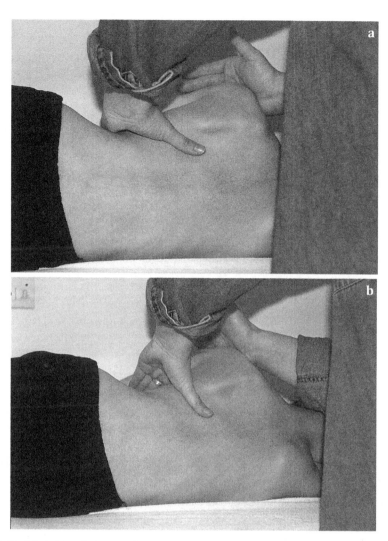

Fig. 7.44: (a) Grip technique and starting point for PEP exercise 2 for thoracic curvature: the cranial correction hand links up with the pisiform bone on the acromion; the caudal hand does the same as in exercise 1. **(b)** Bringing together of the hands.

When performing PEP thoracic exercise (2), the principle is initiated from the same starting position. The pisiform bone in the cranially placed hand contacts the acromion and presses the shoulders against the pressure of the caudally placed hand, in a lateral and caudal direction. The caudally placed hand lies as it did in thoracic exercise (1) and executes the same pressure in the same direction (Fig. 7.44a-b).

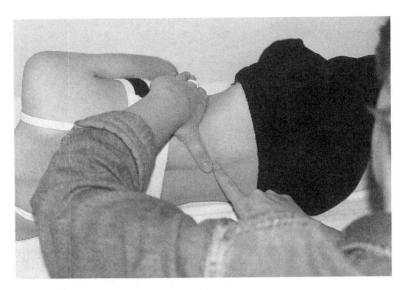

Fig. 7.45: Starting position of exercise 1 for a lumbar curvature. The index finger is pointing to the lumbar apical vertebra.

The PEP program for the lumbar curvature

When performing PEP lumbar exercise (1) the patient lies on the lumbar convex side (Fig. 7.45). The procedure is identical to thoracic exercise (1) in the previous section. The pressure is applied against the lumbar concave side (Fig. 7.46a-b).

When performing PEP lumbar exercise (2) the starting position remains as it was in exercise (1); the hand placed caudally with the pisiform bone contacting the ischial tuberosity and pushes the hip cranially and laterally against the cranially placed hand in the lumbar concavity. The same maneuver with the cranially placed hand is performed as in lumbar exercise (1). The pressure onto the concavities is applied with a slight force vector in a ventral direction and is fitted to the respective torsion behavior of the section of the trunk being treated (Fig. 7.47a-b).

With double curve scoliosis, both curvatures are treated in rotation. With a significant countercurve, one begins with the major curvature and finishes again with the major curvature, with treatment lasting twenty minutes per day, which can be split up into ten minutes in the morning and ten minutes in the afternoon.

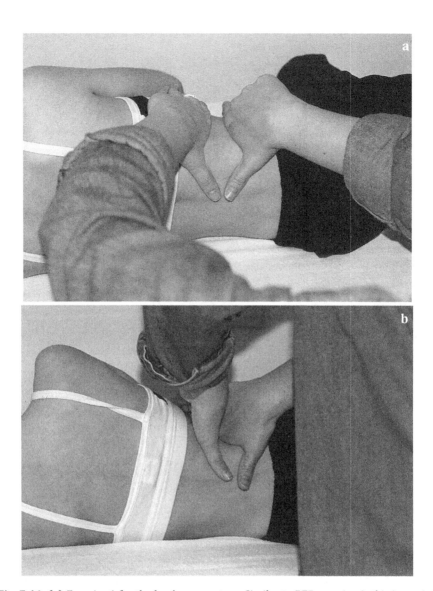

Fig. 7.46: (a) Exercise 1 for the lumbar curvature. Similar to PEP exercise 1, this is carried out for thoracic curvatures. The patient lies on the lumbar convex side and pressure is applied to the lumbar concave side. The hands are again applied in a planar fashion and are kept a certain distance apart. **(b)** Bringing together of the hands with a relocation of the pressure point to the radial side. The direction of the force approaches the apical vertebra.

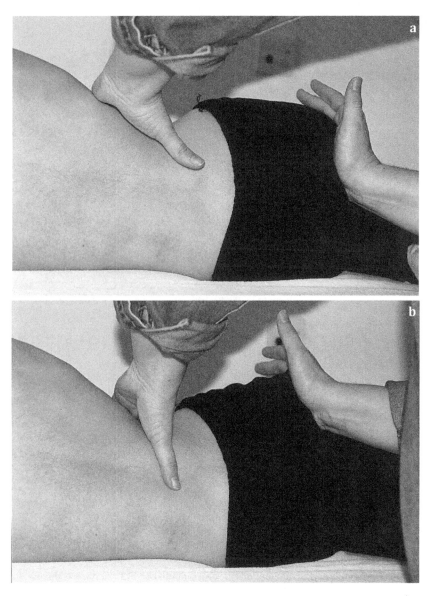

Fig. 7.47: (a) Starting position of exercise 2 for a lumbar curvature. The practitioner's pisiform bone links up with the patient's ischial tuberosity. **(b)** The final position in exercise 2 for a lumbar curvature, from the PEP program. It is held for more than twenty breaths.

The primary responses immediately after treatment with the PEP exercises show that favorable reactions in posture are achieved as a primary effect (Weiss 1993). These primary effects can also be observed with adult patients; however, it can be the case that six to ten sessions must take place before this purely reflex treatment program brings forth responses.

Currently, there are no long-term results for the PEP method. However, it is easy to learn and can be integrated into other treatment systems, meaning it can be considered an enrichment of the therapeutic possibilities in the treatment of scoliosis, particularly in the case of younger children.

7.8 Treatment of decompensated thoracic curvatures with a Cobb angle of more than 70° (Schroth Original System)

Thoracic curvatures greater than 70° Cobb angle without significant lumbar countercurves are usually so rotated that the Schroth Scoliologic® Best Practice program should not be solely relied upon. Sagittally, the thoracic profile appears kyphotic due to the pronounced costal hump. The lumbar profile appears lordotic, partially with a short-arched lordotic curve above the sacrum. This type of scoliosis should be treated according to Schroth's original system. It was with Katharina Schroth's experience when treating such severe thoracic curvatures that she developed her method (cf. Chapter 2.1).

In contrast to treatment of mild idiopathic scoliosis and more severe lumbar curvatures in adulthood, the decompensated thoracic curvature with a Cobb angle greater than 70° is treated like a kyphoscoliosis. For this reason, we have chosen to focus on the most important exercises from Schroth's original system. Further exercises can be found in *Three-Dimensional Treatment for Scoliosis* (Lehnert-Schroth 2007).

However, maneuvers which are applicable to all exercises are a requirement for the exact execution of these exercises. Therefore, a description of these preliminary maneuvers is included. It is assumed that most of these curvatures are right thoracic convex curvatures. In the following descriptions, 'right' always means the side of the costal hump (parcel side) and 'left' always means the weak side.

7.8.1 General correction principles of Schroth's original system

I) The five pelvic corrections

With a functional 3-curve scoliosis, every exercise should contain the five pelvic corrections:

1. Pelvis backwards, as high above the middle position as possible so that the upper body can easily bend forward.

2. If a lumbar lordosis is present, lift the front edge of the pelvis.

3. Shift the protruding hip from the trochanter major in the frontal plane. If the pelvis is in the middle position, this pelvic correction can be omitted.

4. The hip (Ilium) beneath the costal hump is rotated dorsally; the other hip is moved ventrally in order to de-rotate the pelvic girdle as a fixed point against the ribcage.

5. The hip beneath the costal hump is lowered in order to broaden the weak point allowing for increased expansion during inspiration (open) (Lehnert-Schroth 2007).

II) Rotational breathing

Every exercise includes a pelvic correction in combination with rotational breathing; a right angle is cultivated along the flank. The first direction (the first flank) goes in the desired exercise direction; the second flank always goes in a cranial direction, together with the occiput push (neck is along the back).

Every breathing movement occurs in a right angle with an intentionally outwards pointing diaphragm. However, this must first be practiced and felt. The patient should also feel this manually and perceive it emotionally (Lehnert-Schroth 2007).

III) Correction cushion

Correction cushions (approx. 200g bags of rice) are used as a passive correction aid in almost all starting positions, so that the patient is reminded of the untwisting feeling in everyday life and at rest. One must take care that they are placed correctly. When lying on the back, a cushion is placed along the m. gluteus maximus on the thoracic concave side in order to de-rotate the pelvis unilaterally, ventrally. One cushion is placed directly under the shoulder blade on the thoracic concave side, so that not only the shoulder height, but also the entire shoulder girdle is pushed forward on this side. At the costal hump (thoracic convex side), the cushion lies transversely under the scapula so that the ribs located above and below this, as well as the shoulder girdle on this side, can be lowered (Lehnert-Schroth 2007).

IV) Shoulder counter-tension

Shoulder counter-tension and shoulder tension describe the efforts of the patient to push laterally with the shoulders in the frontal plane. The shoulder counter-tension takes place on the thoracic convex side and is the cranial resistance against the costal hump correction in the frontal plane (costal hump medially, shoulder girdle laterally). In contrast, the shoulder tension helps to open the thoracic concave side and thus leads the thoracic shift to the thoracic concave side.

The elbow is bent here and is held at 90°, with the hand encompassing the shoulder on the same side. The elbow pushes laterally (Fig. 7.48 on the right).

V) The occiput push

The occiput push is built into every exercise. The patient wriggles with their spine in the direction of their head, over the neck, and up to the occiput. This creates a feeling of length. The chin is taxed in such a way that one feels like one has a stand-up collar on (Lehnert-Schroth 2007).

VI) The hold-to-twelve exercise

After correction, the best exercise results – identified in the mirror – are securely tensed; that is, the entire trunk musculature is stretched in the correction position, which creates an asymmetric feeling of tension/posture:

a) In the first inhalation phase, the rotational breathing takes place in the weak point in the lumbar region underneath the costal hump. While breathing out, the muscular result is held. When doing this, the patient can also press down on a wooden bar.

b) In each further inhalation, the correction result of the rotational breathing is improved and the air is guided into the thoracic concave side. Subsequently, the trunk muscle tension is repeated in the exhalation phase. Depending on the exercise, two bars can be pushed against the ground during this section.

c) After, the narrow ventral side is moved anterior via the breath and everything is stabilized again. The patient must breathe out with the greatest trunk muscle tension possible, counting to four and with the best correction.

With the next inhalation, the patient corrects again counting to four, and during exhalation the correction position is held under tension. With the third exhalation, the patient counts to four again and, while sitting in a rotated position, for example, the backrest is pulled 'apart' isometrically. After this, the patient will need to rest in a lying position (Lehnert-Schroth 2007).

VII) Rest phases

Rest phases take place in a horizontal position, if possible, without a head cushion, lying on the correction cushions so that the intervertebral discs – which in an upright position experience maximum trunk muscle tension – can fill again. The cushion support should convey a sense of the corrective posture that becomes unconscious through repetition, enabling the untwisting of the trunk section to occur easily in everyday situations (Lehnert-Schroth 2007).

7.8.2 Special correction principles of Schroth's original system

I) The twisted seat (Fig. 7.48)

Starting position: The patient sits with the left half of the pelvis (the pelvis half on the thoracic concave side) on a stool. The right half of the pelvis can overhang laterally to a certain extent (third pelvic correction). The right leg is stretched out behind and rotated outwards in the hip joint. The ankle pushes further in a distal direction (fifth pelvic correction). A correction cushion lies in front of the right half of the pelvis in order to twist it backwards (fourth pelvic correction).

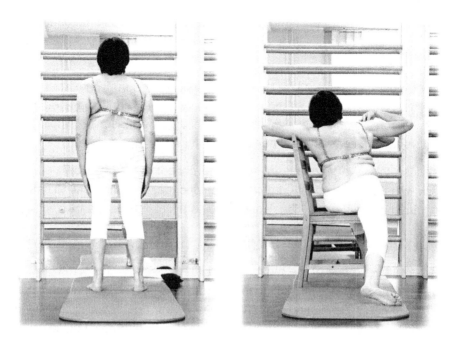

Fig. 7.48: Twisted seat in the execution of exercises with shoulder counter-traction on the right side.

The upper body is obliquely positioned forward as an extension of the leg that is stretched out behind (first and second pelvic corrections result here of their own accord) and slightly to the left. During the execution, both hands press bars into the floor or pull on a fixed bar at the appropriate height. Alternatively, the hands lie on the backrest and push it "apart."

Execution of the exercise begins with the occiput push and opening up of the concave side with a simultaneous broadening of the weak point underneath the costal hump.

a) Weak point (free-floating ribs, right) sideways and cephalad while the diaphragm is lowered. Hold while exhaling. With the next inhalation, the free-floating ribs are forced dorsally and cephalad while lowering of the diaphragm occurs. Hold while exhaling.

b) Weak side is arched sideways and outward while the diaphragm is lowered. This correction is held while exhaling. The same ribs are moved dorsally and cephalad while lowering the diaphragm and held while exhaling.

c) The breath into the right ventral zone is forward and in the direction of the head, always with a lowering of the diaphragm.

d) If the patient is observing themselves corrected in the mirror, the whole body is made "fixed and solid" through isometric tension (twelve tensions). As the patient observes their body corrected in the mirror, during the exhalation (stabilization phase) a whole-body isometric contraction is performed.

Because this is a laborious exercise, the patient should lie down on their back with their legs up on correction cushions that help the trunk to untwist, and run through the exercises once more as a film in their head.

II) The 50x exercise (Fig. 7.49a + b)

This exercise is one of the most important exercises for the correction of a costal hump. The patient sits cross-legged in front of the wooden wall bars; the right knee is cushioned against the nearby bar (fourth pelvic correction). The hands reach for a bar above head height and the patient squiggles up against this with an occiput push so that all concave sections of the trunk are relieved of any load. The constricted, right ventral side of the chest now comes to the front and the patient breathes in a right angle upward (towards the head), which erects the costal hump. While keeping the neck straight, the head is brought as far backward as possible, flattening out the costal hump from above. This can take place over several breaths, making sure to observe the previous correction result during each exhalation.

After correction, the best exercise results – identified in the mirror – are held firmly; that is, the entire trunk musculature is tensed in the correction position, which creates an asymmetric feeling of tension/posture.

As Katharina Schroth saw the effect that this newly developed exercise had with one of her patients, she cried out joyfully, "You must do this exercise 50 times a day!" which is how this exercise got its name.

The patient must carry out the "big arch" for the concave side after this exercise, once the patient has rested in order to complete the untwisting of the upper body (Lehnert-Schroth 2007).

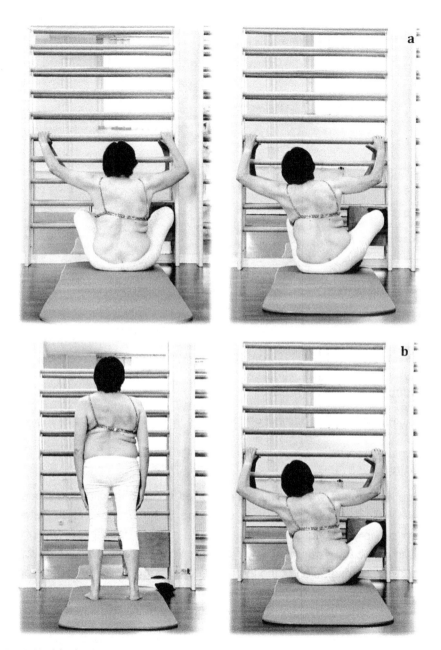

Fig. 7.49: (a) The 50x exercise commences in front of the wooden bars, pushed over to the right on the parcel side (left-hand image). Since the exercise is oriented to the left (right-hand image), one has enough room for maneuver in this manner. **(b)** The 50x exercise in comparison with an uncorrected stance.

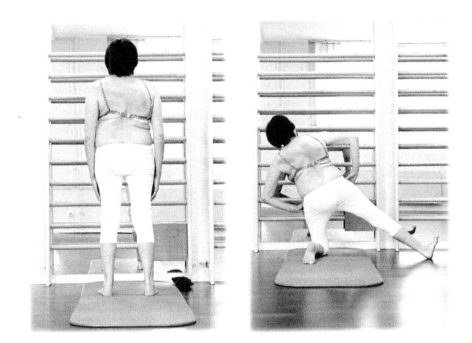

Fig. 7.50: The muscle cylinder in execution, on the knees.

III) Muscle cylinder (Fig. 7.50)

This exercise can be carried out standing, on the knees, or sitting on a stool.

Standing:

The patient stands with the first and second pelvic corrections in place on the left leg. The right leg is in a stretched position and rotated outward (fourth pelvic correction) – the foot is on a stool or resting on one of the wooden wall bars. The upper body is bent slightly forward and a little to the left, making an extension of the leg (third pelvic correction), forcing the right-side waist muscles to support it. The right heel pushes in a distal direction (fifth pelvic correction). This starting position remains unchanged during the exercise.

The rotational breathing is carried out for the right false ribs, the left weak side, the constricted right front side, and the right underarm ribs. Supporting the hip, the left shoulder can sometimes be pulled or pushed too strongly outward/upward, and the shoulder counter-tension is applied simultaneously, on the right-hand side, obliquely outward/backward.

On the knees (see image):

For the exercise, the patient kneels on the left knee. The right leg is straight and rotated outward (fourth pelvic correction). Otherwise, the exercise proceeds as described above.

IV) Door handle exercise (Fig. 7.51a + b)

The door handle exercise is called such because in the beginning, due to a lack of wooden wall bars, Katharina Schroth used a door handle as a hold.

The starting position is kneeling, with the bottom resting on the heels. The patient kneels with their left side facing the wooden wall bars and with the outstretched left arm, grabs hold of the highest bar they can reach above their head. The right lower leg is located roughly five cm behind the other leg in order to untwist the pelvis. The knees are positioned asymmetrically. The right hip (half of the pelvis) is lowered outward and backward (first, second, and third pelvic corrections). The upper body is now positioned obliquely to the left and leaning a little forward (Fig. 7.51a).

The exercise: By bending at the elbow, the left arm pulls the upper body up so that the patient is on their knees while breathing rotationally against the resistance of the untwisted pelvis. The back of the head pulls in the same oblique direction left, until the patient is on their knees. Now the left arm applies resistance while the right hip stretches outward and backward and the arm slowly extends (Fig. 7.51b).

V) The hip knot (Fig. 7.52)

The patient kneels against the third wall bar, possibly with a correction cushion in front of the right knee, which rotates the right pelvis backward (first, second, and fourth pelvic correction). This is also pushed to the right (third pelvic correction).

The hands reach up to a bar above the head. The pelvis is lowered and both sides stretch. The patient performs a slight occiput push upward and to the left. This is the starting position.

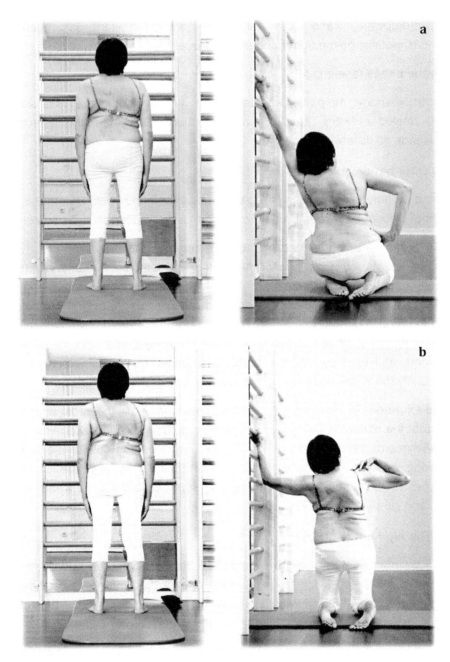

Fig. 7.51: (a) The starting position of the original door handle exercise. **(b)** The finishing position of the door handle exercise.

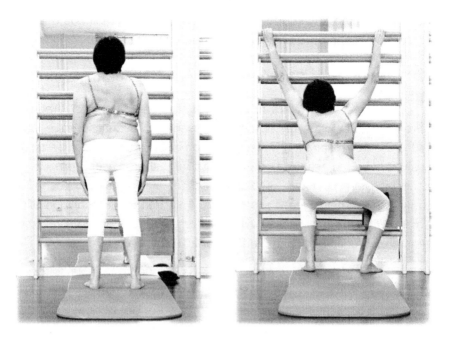

Fig. 7.52: Execution of the hip loop. For comparison purposes on the left: uncorrected in a position of rest.

The exercise: The patient moves the pelvis in a circle, laterally, dorsally, and caudal (fifth pelvic correction), broadening all concave sections of the trunk and filling them via the rotational breathing in each rotation. In opposition, the right side of the chest pulls ventrally in order to diminish the costal hump.

This exercise helps to improve (mobilize) the pelvis correction with stiff functional 3-curve curvatures.

The selection of exercises described here for the treatment of decompensated thoracic curvatures with a Cobb angle greater than 70° are according to Schroth's original system and are sufficient for treating this special pattern of scoliosis. Differences may be observed in the execution of these exercises when compared to the "Power Schroth" exercises, particularly with the door handle exercise, described here.

The rotational breathing technique is simplified with the "Power Schroth" program. The most important consideration is the optimal execution of the exercises, oriented toward the individual, with simplified methods or exactly as described in Schroth's original system (Lehnert-Schroth 2007).

7.9. Biofeedback in Physiotherapy for Treating Scoliosis

The term biofeedback refers to a method that uses technical (frequently electronic) means to make it possible to observe bodily functions (i.e. pulse, blood pressure, respiration, muscle tension, EEG) that cannot be directly perceived by the senses, thereby making them accessible to the consciousness. The focus of biofeedback is akin to that of behavioral therapy and learning theory approaches. This treatment technique allows for many different applications. What is more, it is also used for relaxation during rehabilitation (Rief and Bierbaumer 2011).

Due to the fact that the consciousness is frequently unable to directly perceive the body's own regulatory mechanisms, it is not possible for the senses to be consciously influenced when they are not working properly. A benefit of biofeedback is that it serves to make the consciousness aware of a bodily function by means of physiological measurements. In treating scoliosis, for example, the patient uses this feedback in order to achieve better posture.

More than 100 years ago, devices were already in use for treating scoliosis – partly to support physiotherapy, partly to straighten posture (Fig. 7.53). A few corrective devices were similar to a brace, while others were used as corrective aids for exercises (Schanz 1904, Weiss 2013).

Katharina Schroth introduced a new kind of biofeedback to scoliosis treatment in 1921. Her goal was to achieve the best possible postural correction by using the exercises described. Perception of the best possible posture – "postural consciousness" – was developed by observing visible corrections in a mirror (cf. chapter 2.1). The reflected image enables postural consciousness to be gauged in connection with the current corrective position, with the result that, after a certain amount of practice, the degree of correction can be achieved with certainty in everyday life even without using a mirror to check.

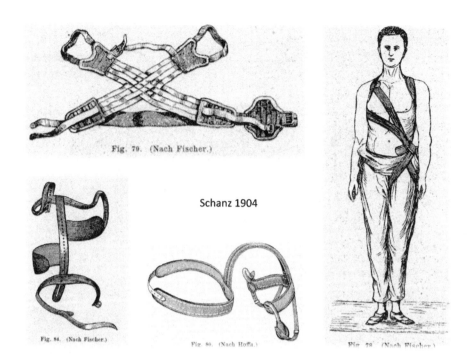

Schanz 1904

Fig. 7.53: Corrective devices, some of them stemming from the 19th century. These were used to straighten posture or in support of physiotherapy and even as braces (Schanz 1904, Weiss 2013).

Although actual biofeedback systems (Rief and Bierbaumer 2011) were first described in the 1980s (Dworkin et al. 1985, Nowotny et al. 1987, Bogdanov et al. 1990, Weiss and Michely 1992, Birbaumer et al. 1994, Wong et al. 2002, Bazzarelli et al. 2002), they have not yet gained acceptance for scoliosis treatment. This is partly because, in the past, wearing the devices involved a great deal of discomfort and partly because rather large units – which had to be attached to the body, were needed for the electronic components (Fig. 7.54).

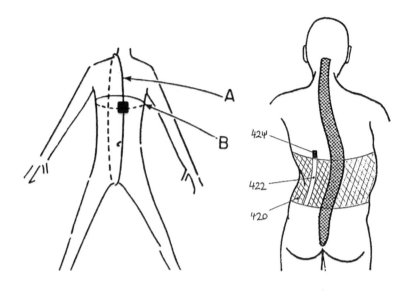

Fig. 7.54: *Left*, schematic drawing of a biofeedback system (modified according to Dworkin et al. 1985). The system was basically used to measure length when treating both scoliosis as well as kyphosis. Discomfort was caused by the location of the longitudinal measurement strap from walking movements and by the placement of the box holding the electronic measuring equipment on the chest. *Right*, schematic drawing of another system designed to measure the concavity of curvature in scoliosis using a sensor (Weiss and Michely 1992).

Tests and methods for improving postural correction based on electromyography were employed for scoliosis treatment in the last century (Weiss 1991, see also Fig. 7.55). Early on, such applications were very unwieldy (Fig. 7.56) due to the large hardware that was required (Weiss 1993). However, today's EMG devices are smaller and more manageable and sometimes do not even require a cable. This allows EMG feedback for gait analysis. So, it is possible that biofeedback for scoliosis may experience a comeback.

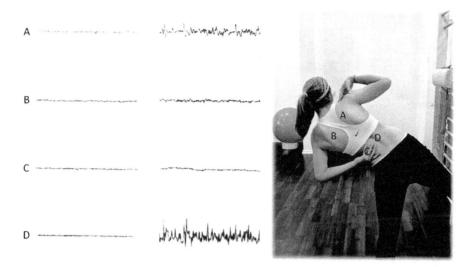

Fig. 7.55: Using EMG in support of targeted physiotherapy. Far *left*, 4-channel EMG in a resting position, recording (A) the thoracic erector spinae (ES) on the convex side at the apex of the curvature, (B) the thoracic ES on the concave side at the apex of the curvature, (C) the intrinsic lumbar portion of the lumbar ES on the convex side in the direction of the fibers, and (D) the intrinsic lumbar portion of the lumbar ES on the concave side in the direction of the fibers. *Center*, activity pattern during the muscle cylinder exercise. *Right*, sample exercise performed for clinical hypercorrection of both lumbar and thoracic scoliosis in patients with right-hand thoracic curvature greater than 50° Cobb (EMG measurements from Weiss 1991). After proper execution of the trunk corrections now head alignment can be improved.

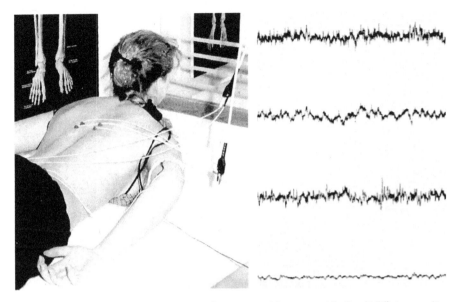

Fig. 7.56: Standardized head-raise test (sensor positions as with Fig. 7.55) to monitor progress during rehabilitation (Weiss 1993).

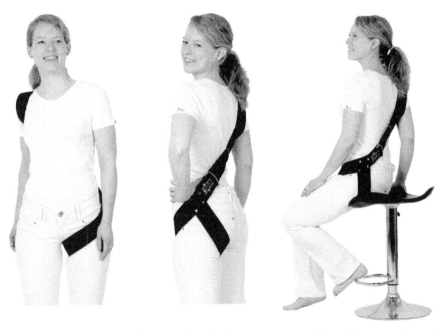

Fig. 7.57: Prototype of the Spinealite® biofeedback system used for right convex thoracic curvature with left convex lumbar countercurvature.

In 2011, a new biofeedback system was developed (Fig. 7.57) using the time-tested corrective principles of the Schroth Scoliologic™ Best Practice program (cf. chapter 7.3; 3D made easy).

The straps of the Spinealite® biofeedback system are partly elastic, so once their tension threshold has been reached (unlike fully elastic belt systems) retention force is maintained, even over months of continuous use.

It is possible to adjust the corrective strength of the system – and thus the tensile strength as well. When ideally adjusted, the system has an excellent corrective effect (Fig. 7.58) that can be substantiated radiologically (Weiss 2013). For slight corrections, the system is hardly noticeable; at its maximum corrective setting, there is a relatively strong pull on the shoulder.

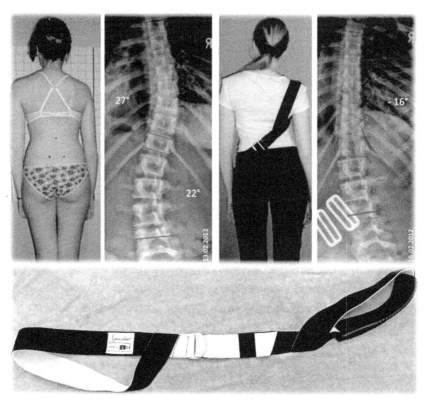

Fig. 7.58: *Top*, hypercorrection effect using the Spinealite® biofeedback system in a patient with adolescent idiopathic scoliosis (AIS) and a thoracic curvature of 27° according to Cobb. *Bottom*, view of the Spinealite® biofeedback system without a patient.

If worn by patients when sleeping at night or when otherwise unconscious, the effectiveness cannot be guaranteed, possibly leading to improper use. That is why, unlike braces, this biofeedback system is intended for patients, when awake, and without limited conscious awareness. This is one reason, we do not refer to it as a brace, which may be worn when sleeping.

The biofeedback character of the system results from an increase in shoulder tension that causes greater wearing discomfort when posture is poor (when the curvature is aggravated). Thus, an aversive stimulus is associated with improper posture, and a pleasant feeling with corrective posture. The more a patient grows accustomed to the corrective pull, the less aware he or she is of the biofeedback response, and increasingly, it becomes a corrective system. Consequently, this system may be used in conjunction with hard-shell braces to provide relief for more pronounced and/or decompensated curvatures, and with the potential for managing physical growth.

When the Spinealite® biofeedback system is used, we recommend initially limiting correction to a range that is easy to tolerate, increasing it every two to three days, or even once a week, until the full corrective effect is reached. This can easily be accomplished independently by patients and/or their parents at home once proper instruction by a competent specialist occurs.

At present, Spinealite® devices are used for up to twelve hours a day during growth spurts to supplement highly corrective hard-shell braces.

If, during the main growth spurt, a patient can not tolerate a hard-shell brace for twenty-three hours a day, he/she can use a Spinealite® device when in school or during recreational activities. Depending on how the Spinealite® is adjusted, this will ensure a certain level of correction even during times when the hard-shell brace is not worn. Benefits of the system are that it is not particularly bulky or conspicuous, and it is flexible. It does not restrict many routine activities and can even be worn during certain sports activities (horseback riding, running, skating, etc.).

Positive feedback has resulted from treating decompensated and painful cases of adult scoliosis as well. When treating adult scoliosis, the goal is to decrease decompensation-induced asymmetric strain on the torso muscles. This is possible even at a slightly corrective setting. By relieving strain, it offers the opportunity to prevent pain. Moreover, proper use of the Spinealite® Biofeedback system reduces the early onset of fatigue during routine activities.

References

Asher MA, Burton DC. Adolescent idiopathic scoliosis: natural history and long-term treatment effects. Scoliosis. 2006;1(1):2.

Bazzarelli M, Durdle N, Lou E, Raso J, Hill D. A wearable networked embedded system for the treatment of scoliosis. Stud Health Technol Inform. 2002;91:383-6.

Birbaumer N, Flor H, Cevey B, Dworkin B, Miller NE. Behavioral treatment of scoliosis and kyphosis. J Psychosom Res. 1994 Aug;38(6):623-8.

Bogdanov OV, Nikolaeva NI, Mikhaïlenok EL. [Correction of posture disorders and scoliosis in schoolchildren using functional biofeedback]. Zh Nevropatol Psikhiatr Im S S Korsakova. 1990;90(8):47-9.

Borysov M, Borysov A. Scoliosis short-term rehabilitation (SSTR) according to 'Best Practice' standards-are the results repeatable? Scoliosis. 2012 Jan 17;7(1):1. doi: 10.1186/1748-7161-7-1.

Burwell, RG. Etiology of idiopathic scoliosis: current concepts. Pediatric Rehabilitation. 2003;6:137–170.

Deacon P, Flood BM. Idiopathic scoliosis in three dimensions: a radiographic and morphometric analysis. J Bone Joint Surg (br). 1984;66-B:509–512.

Ducongé P. Der Skoliotische Flachrücken. Krankengymnastische Therapieansätze. In: Weiss, H.R.: Wirbelsäulendeformitäten (Vol.2), Gustav Fischer Verlag, Stuttgart. 1992, 63–64.

Dworkin B, Miller NE, Dworkin S, Birbaumer N, Brines ML, Jonas S, Schwentker EP, Graham JJ. Behavioral method for the treatment of idiopathic scoliosis. Proc Natl Acad Sci U S A. 1985 Apr;82(8):2493-7.

Farkas A. Über die Bedingungen und auslösenden Momente bei der Skoliose-entwicklung. Stuttgart, Enke 1925.

Glassman SD, Bridwell K, Dimar JR, Horton W, Berven S, Schwab F. The impact of positive sagittal balance in adult spinal deformity. Spine (Phila Pa 1976). 2005 Sep 15;30(18):2024–2029.

Klapp R. Funktionelle Behandlung der Skoliose. Jena: Fischer; 1907.

Klisic P, Nikolic Z. Scoliotic attitudes and idiopathic scoliosis. In: Proceedings of the International Congress on Prevention of Scoliosis in Schoolchildren (Milan: Edizioni Pro Juventute), pp 91–92, 1985.

Lee SG. Improvement of curvature and deformity in a sample of patients with Idiopathic Scoliosis with specific exercises. OA Musculoskeletal Medicine. 2014 Mar 12;2(1):6.

Lehnert-Schroth C. Three-dimensional treatment for scoliosis. The Martindale Press; 2007.

Maruyama T, Kitagawa T, Takeshita K, Mochizuki K, Nakamura K. Conservative treatment for adolescent idiopathic scoliosis: Can it reduce the incidence of surgical treatment? Pediatr Rehabil. 2003 Jul-Dec;6(3-4):215–219.

Mollon G, Rodot JC. Scoliosis structurales mineurs et kinesithérapie. Etude statistique comparative et résultats. Kinésithér Scient. 1986;244:47–56.

Negrini A. Forschungsdaten und ihre Konsequenzen für die Krankengymnastik. In: Weiss, H.R. Wirbelsäulendeformitäten (Vol. 2), Gustav Fischer Verlag, Stuttgart, 85–88, 1992.

Nowotny J, Klyta M, Cieśla T. [Replacement biofeedback in the rehabilitation of children and adolescents with lateral spinal curvature]. Pol Tyg Lek. 1987 Feb 2;42(5):139-43. Review. Polish.

Ozarcuk L. Grundlagen der Skoliosebehandlung mit der propriozeptiven neuromuskulären Fazilitation (PNF). In: Weiss HR (Hrsg) Wirbelsäulendeformitäten Bd. 3, 1994:11–30.

Pugacheva N. Corrective exercises in multimodality therapy of idiopathic scoliosis in children - analysis of six weeks efficiency – pilot study. Stud Health Technol Inform. 2012;176:365–371.

Raso VJ. Biomechanical factors in the etiology of idiopathic scoliosis. Spine: State of the Art Reviews. 2000;14:335–338.

Rief W, Birbaumer N (Editors.): Biofeedback. Grundlagen, Indikationen, Kommunikation, Vorgehen. 3. vollst. überarb. und erw. Auflage. Schattauer, Stuttgart 2011.

Rigo M, Quera-Salvá G, Puigdevall N. Effect of the exclusive employment of physiotherapy in patients with idiopathic scoliosis. Retrospective study. In: Proceedings of the 11th International Congress of the World Confederation For Physical Therapy. London, 28 July – 2 August, 1991: 1319–1321.

Rigo M, Reiter Ch, Weiss H.R. Effect of conservative management on the prevalence of surgery in patients with adolescent idiopathic scoliosis. Pediatric Rehabilitation. 2003;6:209–214.

Schanz A. Die statistischen Belastungsdeformitäten der Wirbelsäule mit besonderer Berücksichtigung der kindlichen Wirbelsäule. Stuttgart: Enke; 1904.

Tomaschewski R. Die Frühbehandlung der beginnenden idiopathischen Skoliose. In: Weiss, H.R.: Wirbelsäulendeformitäten (Vol. 2), Gustav Fischer Verlag, Stuttgart, 51–58, 1992.

van Loon PJ, Kühbauch BA, Thunnissen FB. Forced lordosis on the thoracolumbar junction can correct coronal plane deformity in adolescents with double major curve pattern idiopathic scoliosis. Spine. 2008 Apr 1;33(7):797–801.

von Niederhöffer L. Die Behandlung von Rückgratverkrümmungen (Skoliose) nach dem System Niederhöffer. Berlin: Osterwieck; 1942.

Weiss HR. Elektromyographische Untersuchungen zur skoliosespezifischen Haltungsschulung. Krankengymnastik. 1991;43:361-369.

Weiss HR, Michely A: Meßsystem zur Erfassung der Körperhaltung und von Körperbewegungen, insbesondere als Biofeedback-System. Deutsche Patentanmeldung PA 42 05 790.6. 26.02.1992.

Weiss HR. Imbalance of electromyographic activity and physical rehabilitation of patients with idiopathic scoliosis. Eur Spine J. 1993;1,4:240-243 Mar.

Weiss HR. Frühbehandlung der Skoliose durch peripher evozierte Posturalreaktionen. Z. Krankengymnastik. 1993;4:408–415.

Weiss HR, Lauf R. Contribution to the Etiology of Idiopathic Scoliosis - The "Sobernheim" Concept. In: Proceedings of the Fifth Biannual Conference of the ESDS in Birmingham 1994, 31st May-3rd June 105 - 106.

Weiss HR, Weiss G, Petermann F. Incidence of curvature progression in idiopathic scoliosis patients treated with scoliosis inpatient rehabilitation (SIR): an age- and sex-matched controlled study. Pediatr Rehabil. 2003, Jan–Mar;6(1):23–30.

Weiss HR, Dallmayer R, Gallo R. Sagittal counter forces (SCF) in the treatment of idiopathic scoliosis: a preliminary report. Pediatr Rehabil. 9:1; 2006:24-30 Jan/Mar.

Weiss HR, Hollaender M, Klein R. ADL based scoliosis rehabilitation–the key to an improvement of time-efficiency? Stud Health Technol Inform. 2006;123:594–598.

Weiss HR, Klein R. Improving excellence in scoliosis rehabilitation: a controlled study of matched pairs. Pediatr Rehabil. 2006; 9:3. 190–200 Jul/Sep.

Weiss HR, Seibel S. Scoliosis short-term rehabilitation (SSTR) – A pilot investigation. The Internet Journal of Rehabilitation. 2010;1(1).

Weiss HR. Best Practice in conservative scoliosis care. 4th extended edition, Pflaum, Munich 2012.

Weiss HR, Moramarco M. Scoliosis – treatment indications according to current evidence. OA Musculoskeletal Medicine. 2013 Mar 01;1(1):1.

Weiss HR. History of soft brace treatment in patients with scoliosis: a critical appraisal. Hard Tissue 2013 Jul 01;2(4):35.

Yilmaz H, Kozikoglu L. Inpatient rehabilitation – A systematic Pub Med review. The Internet Journal of Rehabilitation. 2010;1(1).

8 Brace Treatment

The efficacy of brace wear has been confirmed by a number of studies and is supported by a Cochrane review (Negrini et al. 2010) and a recent randomized controlled study known as BrAIST (Weinstein et al. 2013). Scoliosis bracing is an effective, albeit involved treatment, which must be carefully planned and carried out. When fitting a brace, the experience of the orthopedic technician is of immense significance and brace fit should be approved by the attending physician. Brace treatment should be delivered by a team providing a minimum of fifty braces annually and/or under the guidance of an experienced bracing specialist.

With bracing, the end result correlates with corrective effect and wear time. Unfortunately, even with bracing there will still be cases which progress. Brace type is critical and braces vary nationally and internationally. It is up to the brace technician and doctor to ensure the best corrective effect and wearability. It is up to the patient to comply with the recommended wear time for the best opportunity for a positive outcome.

Wearing a brace is necessary if it is suspected that physiotherapeutic measures alone may not be sufficient. This should be assumed in the following cases:

1. When a child shows the first signs of maturation and the angle of curvature exceeds 20°. While it has been stated that eight to ten percent of scoliosis patients may spontaneously remit, this usually only occurs in curvatures of 15° or less in children who are not yet near maturity. With a 20° curvature in a growing child, it is only prudent to assume that a scoliosis will progress unfavorably once the main growth spurt begins. Under this scenario, early treatment at an immature stage is necessary for a beneficial outcome (Fig. 8.1). During this phase, drastic deterioration in scoliosis can occur within a matter of weeks (sometimes more than 30° a year), making growth-channeling measures necessary. It is not uncommon for scoliosis in the high mild to mildly moderate range (20° to 30°) to be able to be corrected significantly at this age, or even

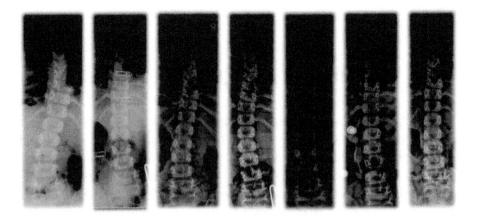

Fig. 8.1: Progression of juvenile idiopathic scoliosis (early onset scoliosis) with a curvature angle of more than 30° at age 6. A continuous reduction in the curvature was attained by constantly wearing a CAD Chêneau brace for approximately sixteen-hours/day. This patient entered the pubertal growth spurt with less than 20° and therefore only required a wearing time of twelve-hours/day during the main growth spurt.

overcorrected, meaning that regular wear of a properly designed, manufactured, and adjusted orthosis may result in significant final corrections. In rare instances, perhaps even curvature straightening may potentially occur after the patient has been weaned off the brace. In other words, for a few, sometimes there is the opportunity to take advantage of a growth spurt to improve a curvature that could increase without a brace. Once menstruation or voice break has set in, the peak of the growth rate is generally past and sustained curvature improvement can no longer be expected in the majority.

2. If a curvature in excess of 20° degrees deteriorates by more than 5° after menstruation or voice break has set in, the scoliosis is categorized as progressive, and wearing a brace to safeguard against expected curvature growth is indicated.

3. When the angle of curvature is more than 30°, full time brace wear is effective up to one year after the onset of menstruation. In cases of delayed bone maturity and curvatures over 40°, full time bracing is often advisable even through the end of the second year after the onset of menstruation.

X-rays are always at the forefront for assessing different treatment strategies. However, an x-ray portrays the spine on one plane only, while scoliosis is, in reality, a three-dimensional deformity with lateral curvature and distortion. When choosing a brace, the patient and family must understand that positive radiological results do not always result in a favorable cosmetic outcome at the conclusion of brace treatment; this is a function of the type of brace selected.

A curvature may appear corrected on the x-ray, but often a rib hump will be visible when observing the spine. In other instances, braces which do not address the sagittal profile can create extremely stiff flatback (Fig. 8.2) which, in itself, can appear visually abnormal. Unfortunately, nonsurgical treatment has sometimes contributed to the formation of flatback. In the

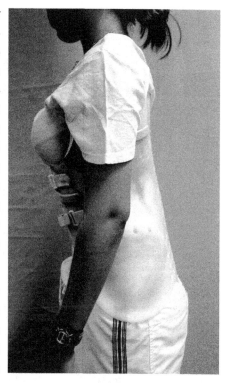

Fig. 8.2: Lateral view of a brace that promotes flatback. The normal sagittal curvatures of the spine are prevented by the brace. Stiffening occurs in an erect position.

past, this problem has plagued more than one brace and the patients who have worn them. Examples are the Boston Brace, and also the German treatment concepts derived from wearing an earlier Chêneau brace (Hopf and Heine 1985). This functional disturbance occurred in spite of well-corrected appearances on frontal plane x-rays.

Numerous bracing concepts (trunk orthoses) are available, but most of them have led to limited treatment success. Unfortunately, skilled orthopedic technicians able to achieve sustainable optimal corrective effects are few and far between.

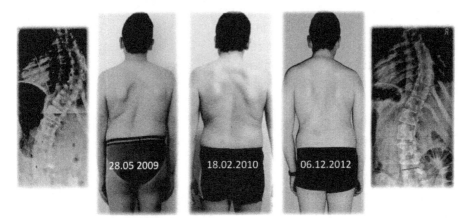

Fig. 8.3: Progression of adolescent idiopathic scoliosis in an adolescent boy with a curvature of 56° at the beginning of brace treatment. Afterwards, the curvature in the x-ray is reduced, markedly compensated, and clinically all but invisible. (From: *Weiss HR, Moramarco M. Remodeling of trunk and backshape deformities in patients with scoliosis using standardized asymmetric CAD / CAM braces. Hard Tissue 2013 Feb 26;2(2):14.*)

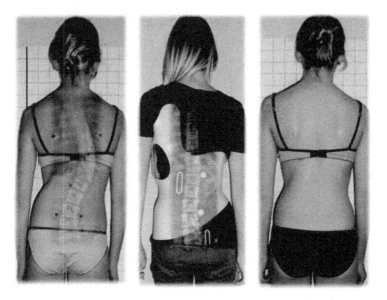

Fig. 8.4: Girl with a right thoracic curve of 42° treated in a CAD/CAM Chêneau brace of the Gensingen library with an intermediate correction in the frontal plane after six months of brace treatment - visible on the *right*.

232

Scoliosis bracing should always be administered by a physician or a specially trained orthopedic technician with an intimate knowledge of the scoliotic spine. When fit properly, the right brace can potentially prevent further trunk deformity and facilitate significant improvements in appearance when the opportunity for residual growth remains.

Most physicians are of the belief that bracing is only effective for curves of 40° or less. However, recently favorable outcomes with curves of greater magnitude are being experienced by those fitted with the Chêneau-Gensingen® brace (Weiss and Moramarco 2013a) (Fig. 8.3). With this Chêneau brace, there is now a reasonable chance to approach clinical corrections achieved as a result of surgery (Fig. 8.4 and 8.5). This newest Chêneau brace is Schroth Best Practice® compatible.

Chêneau was the first brace developer to point out that idiopathic scoliosis of the thoracic spine generally involves flatback and is to be treated accordingly via bracing. For this reason, the most effective Chêneau braces are characterized by how they reproduce the sagittal curvature of the thoracic spine (lateral profile).

The objective of brace treatment is not to straighten the image on the x-ray and dismiss the patient with a case of flatback. As a result, important advances have been made since the time the original Chêneau brace (Fig. 8.6) was developed and this bracing concept has been updated consistently to the point where braces are now able to be produced via plaster-free brace libraries using computer assistance (CAD/CAM). This allows the opportunity for effective correction, for all curve patterns, and the braces created are made expressly for the individual's body based on precise measurements, scans, and consideration of curve pattern. Measurements are then translated into a three-dimensional brace that provides the optimal correction according to each unique curvature.

Designed via CAD/CAM, the Chêneau-Gensingen® brace is also fully compatible with Schroth-based exercise rehabilitation concepts and addresses the trunk in three-dimensions. For the adolescent with scoliosis, this brace strives to address the necessary improvements in trunk deformity, and as a result, halted progression is not its only goal. Due to the comprehensive CAD/CAM library, these advancements in Chêneau bracing are now achievable outside of Germany.

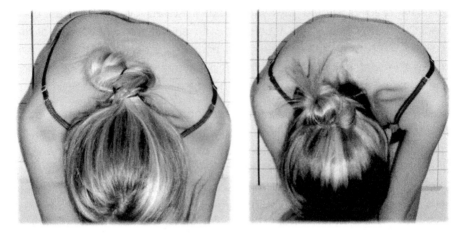

Fig. 8.5: Girl with a right thoracic curve of 42° treated in a CAD/CAM Chêneau brace of the Gensingen library with an intermediate correction of the rib hump - visible on the *right*.

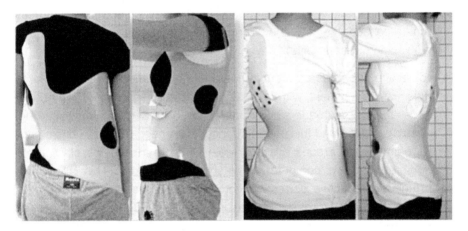

Fig. 8.6: CAD/CAM Chêneau braces (Gensingen brace according to Dr. Weiss / GBW) to treat a double curve pattern. *Left*, from the U.S. (with kind permission from Dr. Moramarco) and *right*, from China (with kind permission from Xiaofeng Nan). The lateral view shows nearly normal sagittal curvature of the spine, rounding in the thoracic spinal area and a hollow in the lumbar spinal area. The arrows show the region of the ventral pressure area.

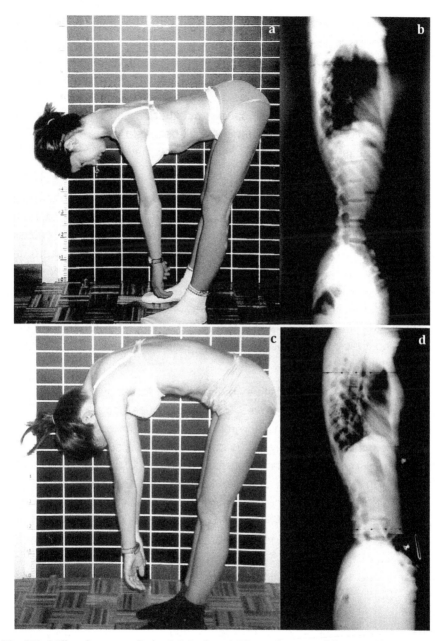

Fig. 8.7: Stiffened extreme flatback **(a)**, also visible on the x-ray **(b)**, caused by improper brace treatment. Below **(c** and **d)**: after twelve months of treatment with a Chêneau brace, nearly normal conditions are observable from the side (modified from Weiss, Rigo, Chêneau 2000).

It has been demonstrated, repeatedly, (Weiss and Moramarco 2013b) that the best cosmetic results are obtainable when, assuming adequate wear time, a significant correction can be achieved when derotation occurs as well. Patients treated with a Chêneau-Gensingen® brace improve appearance of the spinal shape, as seen from the side, and gain improved spinal function. The stiff flatback caused by other brace treatment concepts no longer compares to the functionally well-balanced spine with improved cosmetic results (Fig. 8.7) that patients now have the opportunity to achieve.

Unfortunately, restoring the hollow-back (lordosis) in the lumbar region, which is typically reduced by scoliosis, is often still neglected by most other brace forms as well as other Chêneau derivative braces. This omission occurs, despite our having had the knowledge for several years that restoring the lumbar lordosis can help correct scoliosis (van Loon et al. 2008). Those research results were recently reconfirmed and are accounted for in the design of the Chêneau-Gensingen® brace. Although the Chêneau-Gensingen® successfully addresses the lumbar lordosis, to date, there is no brace which succeeds at correcting the sagittal profile in the thoracic spine.

One of the potential positive outcomes of wearing the Chêneau-Gensingen® brace is improved cosmetic appearance. Patients, and parents, must understand that the recommendation for scoliosis surgery is also for cosmetic purposes, yet, it is often implied that surgery is necessary to reverse curvature to avoid progression and potential cardiopulmonary problems. In truth, there is only a small risk that those with adolescent idiopathic scoliosis, or late onset scoliosis of unknown origin, will ever develop severe cardiopulmonary problems. This is based on the conclusions of a study stating curvatures of 80° to 90° are rarely attained (Asher and Burton 2006). Furthermore, the expectation is that serious problems due to lung function impairment will only occur beyond these levels. Studies cite no substantial increased susceptibility for scoliotics in comparison to a control group of adults without scoliosis (Weinstein et al. 2003, Asher and Burton 2006) with regard to pain for those with late onset scoliosis (initial onset at an age between ten and fourteen years). For these reasons, surgery for scoliosis should be questioned and considered only when the spinal curvature is causing extreme psychological distress or physical impairment. Consequently, brace wear with the goal of improving appearance should be the preferred choice offering far less risk for the patient.

8.1.1 Design variants of trunk orthoses in scoliosis therapy

Corrective trunk braces designed for scoliosis treatment and made from a plaster cast can vary significantly with regard to their quality and effectiveness. In most instances, braces made according to a plaster cast bear the signature of the technician making them. Technicians often specialize in certain curvature patterns and thereby are also capable of attaining outstanding corrective effects for these, yet corrections for alternate curvature patterns may result in an inferior fitting brace. Computer-aided design (CAD) which employs an extensive expert-created database, for all curve patterns, enables quality braces to be manufactured without a plaster cast. Moreover, expert-supported quality assurance serves to mitigate potential sources of error.

| September 2010 | June 2011 | November 2011 | June 2012 |

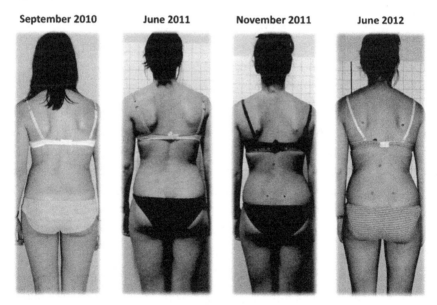

Fig. 8.8: A thirteen-year-old girl with a thoracic curvature of more than 50° at the beginning of treatment with a Chêneau-Gensingen® brace. At the end of treatment, there is good balance and trunk symmetry that reveals almost no sign of scoliosis. (From: *Weiss HR, Moramarco M. Remodeling of trunk and backshape deformities in patients with scoliosis using standardized asymmetric CAD / CAM braces. Hard Tissue 2013 Feb 26;2(2):14.*)

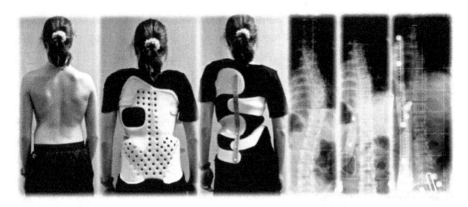

Fig. 8.9: A thirteen-year-old girl with thoracic-type adolescent idiopathic scoliosis of 39° according to Cobb. In the kyphoscoliotic brace, high thoracic 22°, thoracic 12°, lumbar 5°; in the Chêneau light brace, high thoracic 22°, thoracic 8°, and lumbar 11°. In the lumbar area, the corrective force was purposely reduced in order to better compensate the appearance after brace treatment. There was severe pain with the brace in illustration (left brace), which was eliminated after switching to the brace as shown in the *middle* picture.

Today most brace variants neglect to restore physiological or natural lumbar lordosis, even partially. The Chêneau light® brace (no longer available) and the current Chêneau-Gensingen® brace allow for a marked correction of lumbar lordosis that is typically reduced in idiopathic scoliosis (Weiss and Moramarco 2013a).

The design variants now possible for the updated Chêneau-Gensingen® brace have solved the problems other braces encounter and has elevated brace creation to the next level. The Boston brace, as well as other brace variants with an abdominal press, end up aggravating flatback (Danielsson et al. 2007). Flatback is precisely what needs to be avoided as much as possible in light of the assumption that the concomitant loss of a hollow back (in the lumbar spine) favors chronic back pain in adults (Asher and Burton 2006).

Meanwhile, it has been demonstrated that it is not only possible to ably correct scoliosis with higher degree values by using this particular Chêneau brace (Fig. 8.8), but also that successful brace treatment may even approach cosmetic improvements comparable to surgery (Weiss and Moramarco 2013a). However, brace treatment for higher-degree curvatures will only manage to be relatively pain-free if the necessary corrective measures with respect to the lateral profile (i.e. consistent correction of flatback) have been implemented. In the meantime, there is considerable evidence pointing to the fact that the corrective effects of severely painful brace treatment regimens are not forfeited when a non-painful brace providing satisfactory lateral profile correction is used instead (Fig. 8.09).

8.1.2 Corrective effect of the brace

The corrective effect of the brace, previously given in percentage of the initial value, determines the final result within certain limits (Landauer et al. 2003). However, it is necessary to consider the question, "What is the purpose of an outstanding x-ray result if a stiffened flatback ensues, resulting in functional loss and/or pain?"

Furthermore, the following additional questions should be considered: Is it worthwhile wearing the brace if the corrective effect is only slight? How can the percentage of the corrective effect be assessed for major curvatures? Is the radiologic outcome of brace treatment predictible? Is cosmetic improvement possible?

In principle, the corrective effect is of great significance. According to Landauer (2003), at least a 40% primary correction with sustained improvement can be expected, resulting in a 7° correction, on average. Therefore, it stands to reason that, when bracing, the goal should be to constantly exceed this percentage correction to ensure that brace treatment is worthwhile. Of course, not all curvatures are equally correctable. Much depends on the curvature pattern, curvature strength, and individual stiffening. At a curvature of 40°, we sometimes experience overcorrection to −14° (Fig. 8.10). In contrast, sometimes only a correction from 40° to 32° is achieved, despite the fact that braces are designed according to current knowledge, state-of-the-art methods and of superior quality.

The average corrective effect can now be markedly improved even for curvatures with more pronounced stiffening. Accordingly, a well-made and fitted brace is usually effective even when the corrective effect is slight, enabling halting of curvature progression, in most cases, at minimum. Curvatures beyond 60° pose unique challenges and can only rarely be corrected by 50% in-brace. However, with more substantial curvatures, even corrections of less than 40% have led to sustained curvature corrections in individual cases (Fig. 8.11). It is certainly worth considering whether the absolute correction attained, expressed in angular degrees, might not be better suited for establishing a prognosis rather than a percentage correction.

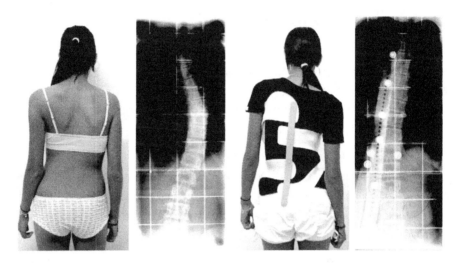

Fig. 8.10: Overcorrection of a thoracic curve of 40° in a Chêneau light brace. The mirroring effect of the brace is also visible on the picture of the patient with the brace on.

Based on clinical experience, a corrective effect of at least 15° should be attained for curvatures beyond the 50° limit in order to stop progression. With a 20° correction and greater, lasting corrections have been achieved, even with curvatures exceeding 50°.

During brace treatment, the problems which sometimes must be solved are not always covered by normal orthopedic or technical orthopedic training. It is necessary that the practitioner have a deep understanding of 3D in-brace corrective movements to avoid compression. The practitioner must also possess the ability to identify challenges and demonstrate the skills needed to solve these stumbling blocks, if and when they appear, after a brace has been fitted or adjusted. Therefore, the Chêneau-Gensingen® brace should be applied at specialized centers, only.

8.1.3 Correction on the x-ray / cosmetic correction

The corrective effect of the brace and the compliance of the patient are two decisive parameters for successful treatment. As long as we measure treatment effectiveness with the x-ray and use the Cobb angle as a parameter for determining success we will wind up with an inadequate view of the overall treatment results. While it is true that Cobb angle is an important measurement parameter, it does not reveal anything with respect to three-dimensional changes or cosmetic improvements.

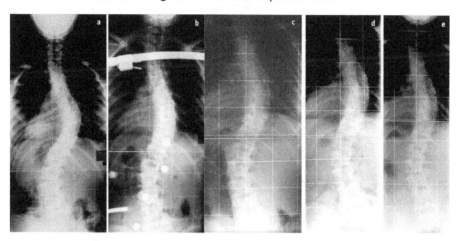

Fig. 8.11: (a) A thirteen-year-old girl with progressive thoracic condition at 62° with qualitatively insufficient initial treatment in December, 1995. **(b)** Correction in the new brace to 46° in January 1996. **(c)** 47°/40° (February 1998); **(d)** 45°/40° (April, 2001) after weaning off the brace and; **(e)** 41°/37° (November, 2002) twenty months after weaning off the brace. The condition was stable, through 2007, six years after weaning off the brace. The patient has gone on to establish her own business and does not feel cosmetically impaired. (Weiss HR (2007) Differentialindikation der Rumpfortheses in der Skoliosebehandlung, MOT 127).

Appelgren and Willner (1990) revealed that many braces tend to aggravate the flatback typically associated with thoracic scoliosis, thus exposing patients to the risk of mechanical functional impairment that in certain circumstances may lead to future complaints.

In current brace variants made according to a precise pattern, the central concern - apart from correcting lateral deviation - is restoration of the normal spinal curvature of the lateral profile. The starting point of the modeling

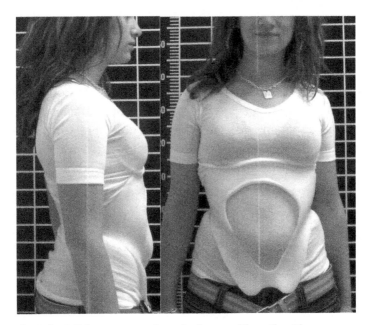

Fig. 8.12: Physio-logic® brace, as seen from the front and from the side.

technique is the idea that it needs to be possible to restore the kyphotic (outwardly round) components in the thoracic area and the lordotic (outwardly hollow) components in the lumbar region. This form must be addressed via the brace. Skilled pressure distribution that only permits kyphotic expansion of the thorax (back rounding) must be successful in restoring the lateral profile without bringing about other cosmetic defects in the thoracic region.

It has been demonstrated that it is possible for a good brace to reestablish kyphosis of the thoracic spine. When treating lumbar scoliosis, the restoration of lumbar lordosis needs to be incorporated in the same fashion as it is typically reduced in such cases.

According to the latest scientific findings, correcting the lateral profile flattened in scoliosis also has a positive effect on lateral deviation and on spinal rotation. This treatment principle has already been realized in the physio-logic® brace, which is able to correct scoliosis of the lumbar spine (Fig. 8.12). This brace can be used when "normal" brace treatment is not possible due to a concomitant disease or a lack of collaboration on the part of the patient. Long-term results for patients during the main growth spurt are not yet available, which is why this brace is only to be recommended when the above mentioned restrictions apply. With that said, this brace has already proven itself in the medium term during growth and in adult scoliosis patients with complaints of pain (Fig. 8.13). Prior to its fitting, the effect of the brace can be simulated by a motion test to find out whether this treatment principle has the potential to be effective for the patient (Weiss 2005).

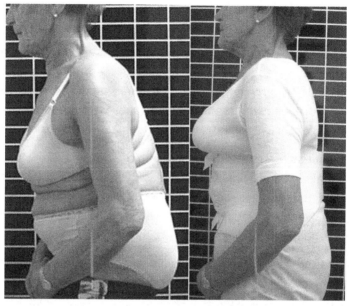

Fig. 8.13: Patient with severe thoracolumbar scoliosis and chronic low-back pain. The physio-logic® brace (first generation) was used to treat her pain. The straightening effect is evident.

8.1.4 Psychological problems related to brace treatment

Wearing a brace during the main growth spurt for twenty-three hours a day may decrease quality of life considerably. This is why very few patients are actually enthusiastic about wearing a brace. If the doctor – patient rapport leaves the patient feeling insecure, it is not surprising that they may ultimately refuse an essential element of treatment participation. Females are frequently hesitant to expose their braces, and so sometimes their wear time unfortunately amounts to no more than sixteen hours, an insufficient amount to gain improvements during the main growth spurt.

However, understanding and empathy usually help to improve the wearing time, especially if the parents manage to maintain composure and deal with issues concerning the brace. Unfortunately, this is not always the case since this situation is frequently unsettling for parents as well as the adolescent. What's more, parents often feel guilty ("How could this have happened?") and are now looking for the 'best way" to treat their children "as quickly as possible."

The parent must exercise caution in this instance. Inquiries are made to all types of practitioners, including those marketing heavily on the internet. This leads to uncertainty and added stress for families due to the opinions of self-proclaimed experts who are not necessarily trained scoliosis professionals or those who are using techniques which lack documentation or a record of success. The result for families is added confusion and doubt.

The mental stress that children and parents are subjected to when making decisions sometimes requires psychological support. In very few cases are the fears and self-reproach justified. In fact, such feelings are by no means a solid foundation for the necessary decision-making process and may even prevent treatments from attaining their potential for success.

It is clear that brace treatment compromises the quality of life of those who wear them, which is why it is not only important for specialists to incorporate the latest technical advances in their work, but also to work to advance brace treatment. Efforts must continue until it is established, with certainty, that quality of life impairment is offset by successful treatments – treatments that reliably avert surgery and result in a satisfied patient.

8.1.5 Learning to wear a brace

In some braces, major problems and discomfort may occur. This is the reason that patients are often advised to get accustomed to wearing a brace slowly. Fortunately, the recent CAD/CAM developments usually result in a brace which can be worn full time from the start.

Once the initial fitting and adjustments for improving the wearing comfort of the Chêneau-Gensingen® brace have been administered, it should be worn as regularly as possible, immediately, and throughout the main growth spurt. To relieve pressure as necessary in a minority of patients, it is sufficient to simply open the clasps of the brace for 15–20 minutes and then re-tighten them. These periods of rest allow the skin to recover, thus enabling the body to frequently tolerate an uninterrupted wearing time of more than twenty hours, even on the first day. Generally, after about a week of brace wear, the brace should then be tolerated for twenty-three hours daily. However, if there is any difficulty sleeping while learning to wear the brace full-time, it is recommended to wait three days before attempting to wear the brace at night again. Otherwise, the loss of sleep from repeated attempts, night after night, can have a demoralizing effect.

When the patient is adjusting to brace wear, any complaints should be taken seriously. It is extremely important to recognize and eliminate problems so that at the end of the introduction period, the only pressure still felt is at the necessary pressure points.

If the truss pad covers a large patch of skin around the main pressure areas, then a good corrective effect will be achieved with a minimum amount of physical impairment. Pain occurs if there is no clearance (voids) in the brace for the corrective movement to take place. The lack of such clearance squeezes the trunk, which is not generally tolerated well. The solution to this problem does not come from reducing the pressure (and thus diminishing the corrective effect), but rather by addressing the lack of clearance areas via increased space. Unfortunately, the clearance areas make the brace a little bulkier, but this is precisely the way to achieve the best effect. Should there still be pain after any problems have been eliminated, it will be necessary for the patient to be re-examined. In individual cases, rib blocking may prevent the brace from being tolerated. In such instances, physiotherapy, manual therapy, or chiropractic manipulation should be sought to reduce the pain caused by movement issues; medications and massages, medicinal baths, electrotherapy, or simply rest may also be prescribed if there is costovertebral joint inflammation.

Another part of the process of brace adjustment is for the practitioner to provide extensive information and answers to every question. Patients often attend the consultation sessions with their parents. If, in the course of the conversation and examination it is evident that the parents may react emotionally, it is advisable for the attending doctor to speak with them alone and present the issues in a disarming manner. In certain cases, remarks made by the parents could potentially result in the child declining the necessary brace treatment or viewing it as something awful. At the same time, the attending physician should not exert pressure, but rather allow the child or adolescent to be responsible for making the decision on his or her own as much as possible. Showing understanding and providing ample information is usually more than sufficient to awaken a sense of personal responsibility, even in children under ten years of age. This acceptance helps contribute to a favorable course of treatment.

On the other hand, during the course of early treatment, parents who are overzealous must not admonish their child regarding time in the brace since during this phase of personality development it might foster resistance and result in outright refusal to wear the brace. It is far better for the child to successfully become accustomed to brace wear on their own terms, even if it is fourteen days into the future, rather than rejecting the brace from the onset.

At the beginning of the wearing phase, it is sometimes necessary to treat the pressure points of the skin by brushing them and applying rubbing alcohol. Creams should be avoided, as they soften the skin, thereby making it less resistant to pressure. A slight reddening of the skin is normal at the beginning of brace treatment.

The Chêneau-Gensingen® brace is standardized and fine-tuned to such an extent that the above-described skin care usually only needs to be recommended when treating curvatures beyond the 60°. Skin irritations occur infrequently in curves below 60°.

8.1.6 Treatment duration and weaning off the brace

Treatment duration can vary widely. Should the wearing-in period of the brace result in completely correcting or even overcorrecting a relatively slight curvature angle, it may well be that the process of weaning off the brace can be started after the onset of menstruation – before a marked curvature in the opposite direction ensues. For more pronounced scoliosis curvatures (approximately 40°) which typically do not correct as well as curves under 40°, it is necessary to wear the brace for as long as possible. In the past, girls almost always weaned from the brace at fifteen or sixteen years of age. It has been demonstrated that longer wearing times lead to better (cosmetic) results with the Cheneau-Gensingen®. This can probably be attributed to the fact that spinal growth still continues to some small degree for more than two years after the growth plates visible on the x-ray have closed. With more pronounced curvatures, e.g. 60° or more, weaning off the brace at age sixteen is not usually recommended. Typically, it is best to begin weaning closer to eighteen to twenty years, depending on the state of maturity.

Braces worn full time may be taken off for school sports. However, the brace should be put back on again immediately after sports participation so the wearing time is not reduced unnecessarily. Competitive sports should mostly be avoided by scoliosis patients with a brace if it could cause the spine to become hypermobile. This does not rule out deciding in favor of competitive sports in individual cases (e.g. swimming).

Should problems surface when wearing a brace, such as pain, tingling sensations, or even nausea and shortness of breath, the attending practitioner should be consulted. The cause can be determined and then any technical problems addressed. For technical problems with the brace (torn off clasp, cracked frame, etc.), the fitting technician should be consulted.

X-rays are necessary for checkups and result in a certain amount of radiation exposure. In slender persons, this can be reduced by taking x-rays with the brace on (1) with half of the exposure time and (2) by reducing the field of exposure to the region of interest (ROI) as described by Weiss and Seibel (2013). In thin children, when exposure time is reduced by half, all details of the bone structure are still recognizable (Fig. 8.14). Even an overlay of the radiation field on the curvature area allows the radiation exposure to be reduced considerably (Weiss and Seibel 2013).

For the trunk muscles to become accustomed to being without the brace, it is necessary for gradual weaning from the brace to take place at the treatment conclusion. To do this, wearing time is reduced by 3-4 hours a day for a period of three months after which the brace is only worn at night for the final six months.

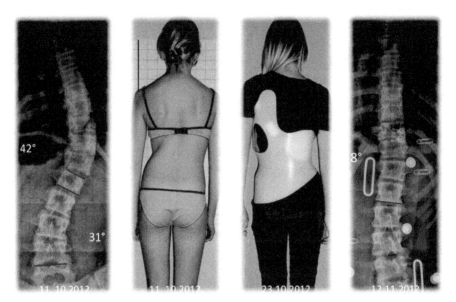

Fig. 8.14: Patient with scoliosis and vast progression in the short-term, prior to brace treatment, with x-rays taken in accordance with the least possible exposure to radiation. The region of interest (ROI) is clearly visible and even with a reduction of the exposure time, the structural entities of the bony tissue are visible.

8.2 Frequently Asked Questions (FAQ) – What Can Patients Expect from Bracing?

Brace treatment for patients with scoliosis can be regarded as a long-lasting impairment of quality of life and therefore a great challenge. To undertake this task, the patient needs to be informed not only about the realistic aims of treatment, but also about problems arising from the spinal deformity itself. It is only under this precondition that the patient can decide about brace treatment and take responsibility for treatment.

The objective of this section is to address the most important issues involved with brace treatment. Addressing these issues is beneficial for the professionals who regularly treat patients with scoliosis and is necessary since there are so many inappropriate and scientifically unacceptable claims and false statements made on the Internet. For example, it is necessary to minimize the fears of the patients and their families when preconceived notions dictate that a brace must be painful to wear to be effective. This is categorically untrue.

Answers concerning the percentage of an in-brace correction cannot be reduced to a simple number. This may cause uncertainty in patients and their parents, although there will sometimes be a beneficial outcome even with an in-brace correction of less than 50%. However, a true professional will not be satisfied with an in-brace correction of 50% when the curvature will easily permit a far greater amount of correction. Of course, the best possible in-brace correction is not worth anything if the patient is not compliant with brace wear.

The following is a brief list of questions that arise on a daily basis in the practice of a conservative scoliosis specialist, followed by the appropriate answers which are based on scientific evidence.

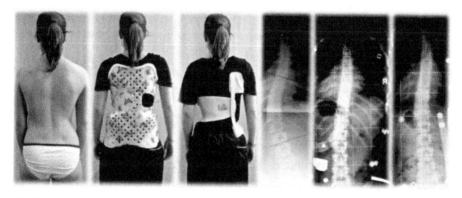

Fig. 8.15: Excellent corrective effect in a "compression brace" that was not able to be worn due to pain (to the *left* in the picture). The Chêneau light® brace achieved the same degree of correction and was able to be worn for twenty-three hours a day, *right* (see also Scoliosis 2010, 5:19).

1. Is brace treatment painful?

A good brace corrects the deformity to the best possible extent without causing pain. An actual correction can only take place when there is room for the corrective movement, not by applying compressive forces.

Sometimes the corrective effect of compression braces can be satisfactory, but this correction is pointless if the brace cannot be worn due to pain. An unpublished study from Stuttgart (Germany) investigating the use of compression braces by a sample of scoliosis patients showed excellent in-brace corrections; however, 50% of the patients dropped out of the study because they were not able to wear the brace, thus making this study unproductive (Fig. 8.15).

2. What degree of in-brace correction can be expected?

We strive for a 50% reduction in-brace, but due a variety of factors, this is not always achieveable. In-brace correction is dependent upon the patient and the individual brace.

Patient-dependent factors:
- Curve pattern
- Patient age
- Curvature stiffness
- Capability of the patient
- Compliance

Brace-dependent factors:
- Pattern specificity
- Shifting of the trunk areas against each other
- Exact fit

Double or triple curve patterns allow far less correction than single curve patterns. The curve of an eleven-year-old girl can be corrected more easily than the curve of a sixteen-year-old girl with comparable Cobb angles and comparable curve patterns wearing the same brace type.

According to recent scientific findings (Weiss 2007, 2011) the in-brace correction should exceed 15°; however, in stiff curvatures this is not always possible (see Fig. 8.16–8.19). Nevertheless, a true professional will not readily accept a low in-brace correction. When the pattern of curvature in the brace is obviously not corrected, the lack of in-brace correction may not be due to curvature stiffness. However, when a brace is designed according to the current "state-of-the-art" standard and improvements to the brace do not lead to an increased in-brace correction it can be attributed to the stiffness of the curvature (e.g. tethered cord). Only the experienced specialist will be able to distinguish between these facts.

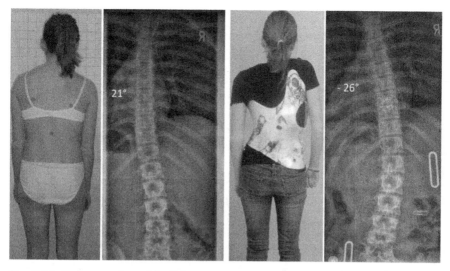

Fig. 8.16: Overcorrection with slight curvature in a premature girl. If good compliance brings the curvature well below the 20° limit by the next checkup, part-time treatment may be possible (12–16 hours), even though menstruation has not yet commenced. The best possible correction can now involve a treatment duration which is as short as possible (see also Scoliosis 2010, 5:22).

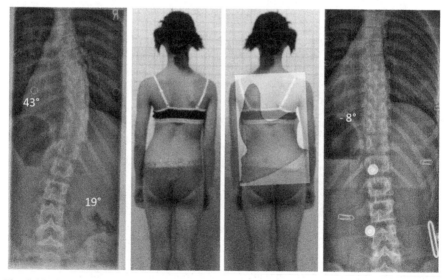

Fig. 8.17: Overcorrection of a curvature of > 40°. This correction allows for the prospect of an excellent final result. The CAD planning can be seen in the middle, along with the brace model on the right of the x-ray, in the 3CH Chêneau-Gensingen® brace (see also Scoliosis 2010, 5:22).

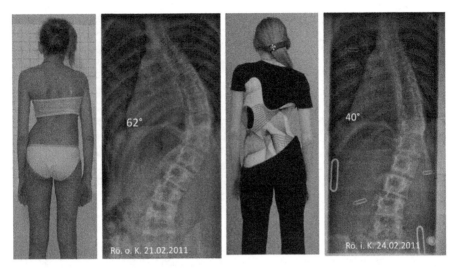

Fig. 8.18: Good re-compensation of a very severe and rigid curvature. The mirror effect is visible. There is the prospect of a markedly improved cosmetic result (see also Scoliosis 2010, 5:22).

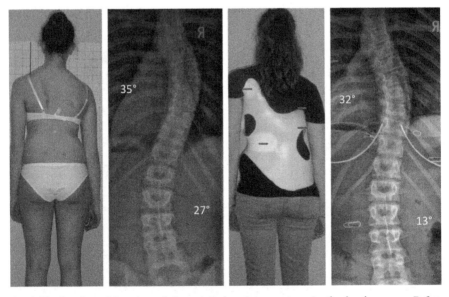

Fig. 8.19: Good straightening of the original main curvature in the lumbar area. Before treatment was initiated, the thoracic curvature was progressive during the previous growth spurt in the patient's first brace and no longer able to be rectified for this patient, now fifteen- years-old. The brace did not offer any further possibilities for improvement (see also Scoliosis 2010, 5:22).

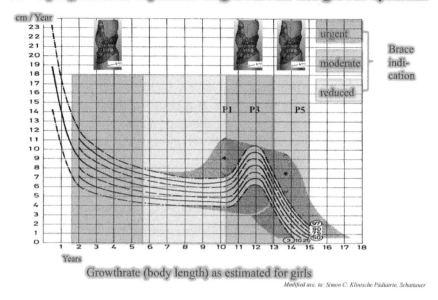

Curve progression is dependent on growth rate and growth dynamics

cm / Year

Years

Growthrate (body length) as estimated for girls

Modified acc. to: Simon C: Klinische Pädiatrie, Schattauer

Fig. 8.20: The growth curve for girls: Between age six and the onset of the first signs of maturity, there is generally no significant increase in curvature. Once the first signs of maturity ensue (P1), a considerable increase in curvature can be expected. Depending on the severity of the curvature, timely brace treatment may be necessary since an increase in curvature can occur within only a few weeks during the main growth spurt.

3. Do I need to be braced with a curvature of 20°?

This question can only be addressed when a wider range of facts are taken into account. For example, a seven-year-old child usually has not yet reached the pubertal growth spurt (Fig. 8.20) and, therefore, does not yet require a full-time brace, but may benefit from nighttime bracing. Likewise, a sixteen-year old girl with the same 20° curvature usually has no further residual growth and does not necessarily require brace treatment. However, an 11-year-old girl with a 20° curvature, according to current knowledge, needs full-time bracing because she is in the pubertal growth spurt, is at 80% risk for being progressive and has the opportunity for final correction with the Chêneau-Gensingen® brace (Fig. 8.16 and 8.17).

If a patient is braced at an early stage and achieves an acceptable in-brace correction, there is a good chance for brace wear time to be cut back early if the curve is below 15° after 6 months of brace treatment. This is not as easily achieved in more mature patients with larger angles of curvature (Fig. 8.18 and 8.19).

During the pubertal growth spurt, curvatures of 15° should also be braced at least part-time, especially when there is a large deformity in comparison to the Cobb angle (large rotation, slight lateral deviation). In such a case, if no treatment commences, an unfavorable prognosis can be assumed.

4. What can be regarded as successful brace treatment?

When the Cobb angle of a curve at high risk of progression is kept stable within the limits of the accepted measuring error (+/-5°) until growth ends, this is regarded as successful brace treatment. For the Boston brace, the success rate appears to be 70%, and for the old Chêneau brace (1999 standards), 80%. Recent publications show the success rate of the CAD/CAM Chêneau brace (Gensingen library) is over 95% for the skeletally immature (Weiss and Werkmann 2012). In curvatures between 20 and 40°, a final correction of the curve and deformity may be achieved when the brace is worn full time during residual growth (Fig. 8.21–8.23.).

Nevertheless, even in patients of relative maturity and with little residual growth remaining, cosmetic improvements (e.g., a recompensation of the trunk) can be achieved using braces from the Gensingen library. Such cosmetic improvements significantly reduce deformity-dependent stress that the patient might experience and thereby reduce the desire to undergo surgery.

Unfortunately, even patients being treated with the best brace may quit brace wear. In addition, growth dynamics are unpredictable and sometimes the brace – initially adjusted properly – is unsuitable at a checkup due to patient growth. When it is decided at the checkup to leave the brace as is or with minor corrections for another three months and the patient grows drastically, in rare instances the curvature can increase because of the fast growth and unpredictable growth timing (growth peak at the wrong time). A combination of factors could result in the brace becoming unsuitable; yet, braces cannot be renewed too often due to cost.

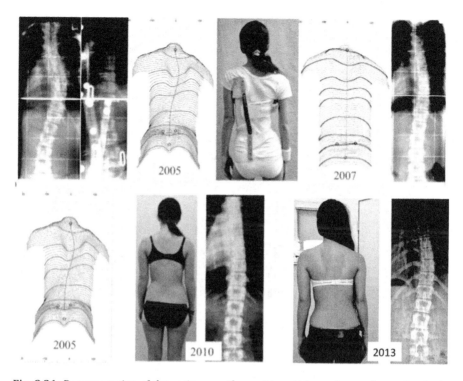

Fig. 8.21: Documentation of the entire growth spurt in a Chêneau brace: Correction in the brace from 38° to - 14°, interim result 19° after two years, final result 14° at eighteen months after weaning from the brace (2010). Visually, no change with a Cobb angle of 19° at a five-year followup without a brace (2013). In this patient both radiological evidence and clinical straightening were possible (see also Scoliosis 2010, 5:19).

Finally, a significant end-result correction, as seen on x-ray, can only be achieved in patients with significant residual growth and full-time brace wearing time (Weiss and Moramarco 2013a). In more mature individuals (girls of fourteen, and boys of sixteen-years-old), residual progression may easily be stopped and an improvement to the clinical aspect (cosmesis) is possible. However, as with improvements as a result of surgery, long-term data is lacking and there is no evidence validating that improvements achieved via bracing can be regarded as stable in the long term.

In curvatures beyond 40°, significant and stable improvements persisting five years after brace weaning seem to be rare; however, progression can be stopped in most of these cases using recent CAD/CAM-based Chêneau derivatives (Fig. 8.24).

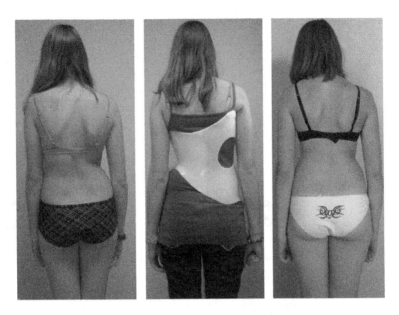

Fig. 8.22: Clinical improvement after only six weeks of full-time wear (see also Scoliosis 2010, 5:22).

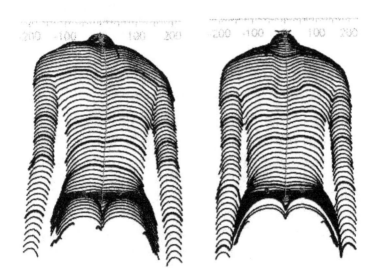

Fig. 8.23: Clinical improvement on surface reconstruction within two years of brace treatment in a patient with a curve of 36° at the start of treatment. The patient remained stable after two years without a brace. The obvious visual decompensation was able to be eliminated.

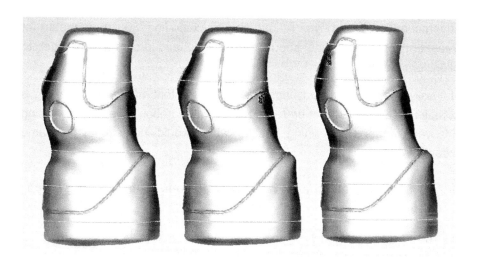

Fig. 8.24 *Left:* Computer model of a brace for treating three-curve scoliosis (see also Figs. 8.17 and 8.18) of version "Chêneau-Gensingen Brace®" V2.03. *Middle:* Increasing the shift to the left (lateral shift). With this change, a noticeable "lump" appears in the middle picture on the left-hand side. *Right:* By straightening the upper body (shifting this molded part to the left), the lump becomes relatively smaller, yet the shift can be left as is. This is an example of how braces can be further developed in the future. It is quite simple to solve these issues for certain brace types by computer and eliminate them once and for all. This results in an excellent corrective effect, but at the same time also ensures wearing comfort.

5. How long will it be necessary to wear the brace?

The main indication for brace treatment as a growth-channeling treatment is during growth phases. During the main growth phase, a progression of 20° to 30° may occur within a few weeks in a non-braced patient. At the end of the pubertal growth phase (fifteen years of age in girls and seventeen years in boys), progression exceeding 15° within a single year will not usually occur. However, the professional must bear in mind that even at the end of the pubertal growth spurt, significant improvements to balance and clinical appearance are possible with treatment via the Schroth-based Best Practice brace. Brace treatment may also be important at this juncture to improve patient collaboration and reduce the patient's desire to undergo surgery.

In a compliant patient with a curvature of less than 30° at the initiation of treatment, weaning can usually begin at the age of fifteen years in girls and seventeen years in boys. In curvatures exceeding 30° at the start of treatment, brace weaning should be delayed and prolonged in order to allow for stabilization.

Naturally, the curvature may increase to some extent after brace weaning is complete. This should not be regarded as deterioration. Even when waiting one year longer for weaning, the curvature would increase to the same extent.

6. *Is it necessary to undergo rehabilitation continuously during brace treatment?*

As discussed previously, physiotherapeutic instruction may have a beneficial effect on patients with scoliosis when applied curve-pattern-specifically. Nevertheless, during growth, the effect of brace treatment should be regarded as the primary treatment method (Fig. 5.2). In children and adolescents under brace treatment, there is no reduction in muscle activity while wearing a brace.

Rehabilitation instruction at certified centers can provide psychological support and help embolden the patient during brace treatment. Obviously, effective, corrective, evidenced-based conservative measures which share correlating principles may be helpful and contribute to an improved outcome at skeletal maturity; however, if physiotherapeutic approaches create undue stress, use of an effective brace, at minimum, should be the first recommended approach during the pubertal growth spurt.

At brace weaning, it is advisable to step up Schroth Best Practice rehabilitation instruction to reinforce concepts which show how to avoid postures which may increase the curvature and overload the spine during daily activities. Intensive treatment based on curve-pattern and curve severity should be prescribed if rehabilitation instruction has never previously occurred.

8.3 Future developments in brace treatment – a perspective

With the advent of CAD technology, it has become possible to reinforce the corrections to the limit of what is tolerable (Fig. 8.24). However, more pronounced trunk displacement is a consideration and can be conspicuous and keep the adolescent from wearing such a "lopsided" brace at school.

Possible future prospects might be a combined application system (Chêneau-Gensingen® and a biofeedback device). Application of this combination might incorporate maximum-correction treatment for eight to twelve hours wearing the hard brace in conjunction with a flexible correction biofeedback type device that the patient might use in daytime that is not obvious during school and leisure activities. Unfortunately, the systems (soft braces) introduced to date are not suitable for a wide variety of reasons.

As a result, the first author has developed a new biofeedback system mentioned in the last chapter, based on the most recent levels of scientific knowledge (Weiss 2013).

This device is relatively simple to apply. It cannot be considered as comfortable, however, since the correction occurs through traction on a shoulder. Wearing comfort also changes subject to the traction force set (correction). For adolescents, the maximum set correction may entail sacrifices in comfort.

Positive results have been experienced with a milder correction traction in adults with severe curvatures. With this scenario, it is not a question of maximum correction, but rather, preventing the trunk from drifting off to the side, which, when occurring over the course of the day often leads to pain and fatigue.

The corrective effect of this system has already been demonstrated (Fig. 7.58). Long-term results, however, are not yet available.

8.4. Brace Treatment for Non-Idiopathic Scoliosis

Most reports of brace treatment involve patients with idiopathic scoliosis. Minimal information is available regarding the effects of bracing on symptomatic and syndromic cases of scoliosis (see also Chapter 1).

Symptomatic scoliosis and/or syndromic scoliosis (Winter 1995) usually has an unfavorable prognosis with brace treatment, except in the case of balanced formation defects which often do not require treatment with a brace.

According to current findings regarding scoliosis surgery, medium and long-term complication rates are high and evidence for surgery is lacking (Bettan-Saltikov et al. 2013; Cheuk et al. 2014). As with idiopathic scoliosis, conservative treatment measures must be considered in cases of symptomatic scoliosis and/or syndromic scoliosis.

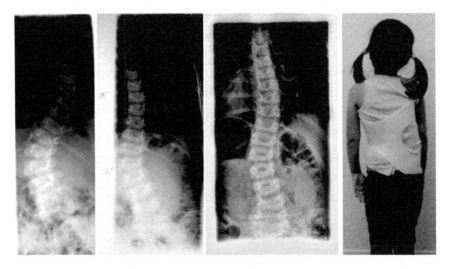

Fig. 8.25: A 2-year-old girl with Marfan syndrome who was brought to the first author with a double major curvature and a Cobb angle of 20°. At first, the course of the condition was observed. Within 6 months, there was progression to a Cobb angle of 50°. Right away, specific CAD/CAM Chêneau brace treatment was initiated. Through consistent treatment with this method, the curvature was reduced to a Cobb angle of 24° without the brace at the age of 4.6 years.

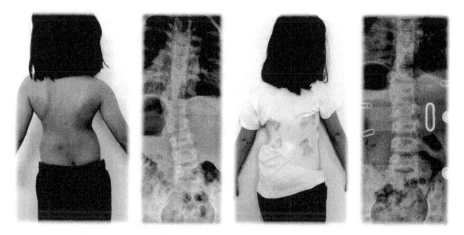

Fig. 8.26: Good corrective effect in a small patient with a congenital formation defect (thoracolumbar hemivertebra).

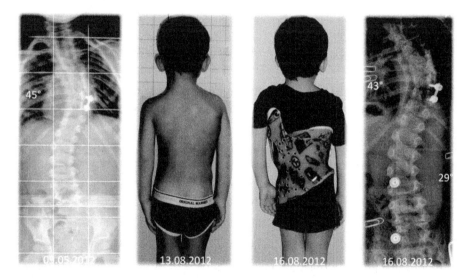

Fig. 8.27: Boy with progressive congenital scoliosis after an operation who was originally fitted with a CAD/CAM brace with a corrective effect in order to find out whether a partial correction would cause a complication in the postoperative condition. This treatment did not result in any complications; however, the curvature increased, but halted clinically (ATR improved) by means of Gensingen brace treatment offering a pronounced shift.

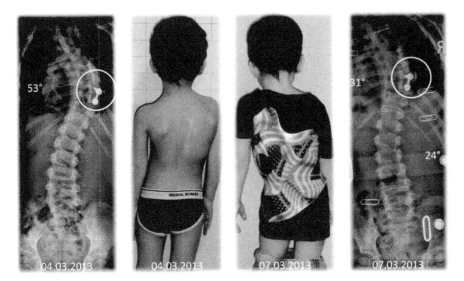

Fig. 8.28: Second brace for the boy in Fig. 8.27. This treatment initially halted the progression. The first brace with less correction did not create complications so we applied the full corrective movement in the brace with a reasonable in-brace correction (compared to 8.27).

Due to the scarcity of individual clinical information accompanying the less common types of congenital scoliosis, little comprehensive research has been conducted to study how patients are affected by conservative treatment. One reason for the scarcity may be that symptomatic scoliosis and/or syndromic scoliosis is often operated on at an early stage – in spite of the uncertain outcomes. There are a few encouraging case descriptions of brace treatment (Fig. 8.25) in patients with an unfavorable prognosis and documented progression before the beginning of treatment (Weiss 2012).

The corrective results from braces according to the current CAD/CAM standard are not as significant with congenital scoliosis when compared to idiopathic scoliosis (Fig. 8.26). Also, with congenital scoliosis, there are still cases which are progressive following surgery.

The question is whether the newest corrective brace treatment should generally be the first treatment approach before a surgical intervention occurs. Figures 8.27 and 8.28 are illustrations/photos of a young boy with progressive congenital scoliosis after surgery. At first this boy was fitted with a low corrective CAD/CAM brace in order to determine whether a partial

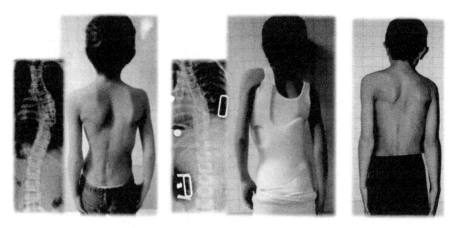

Fig. 8.29: Boy with severe scoliosis deformity in conjunction with neurofibromatosis. Clear decompensation of the thoracic curvature to the right. Clearly visible clinical correction in the USA-produced Chêneau-Gensingen® brace (Scoliosis 3DC).

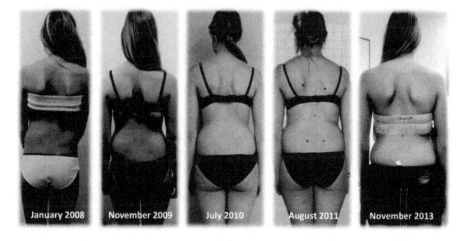

January 2008   November 2009   July 2010   August 2011   November 2013

Fig. 8.30: *Left*: immature girl with a decompensated thoracic curvature and a high risk of progression. Other photos show improvement over the course of treatment with specific Chêneau braces and, as of 2009, with the Gensingen brace. Clear recompensation resulted in an improved postural appearance after complete maturation, even without full compliance.

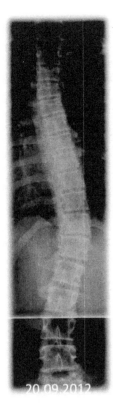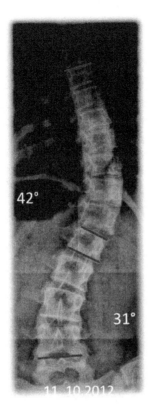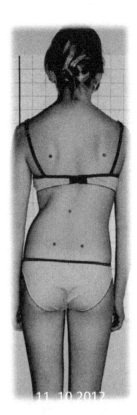

Fig. 8.31: Fast progression in an immature 15-year-old girl within 3 weeks. The curvature increased 20° while she waited for an appointment at the office of the first author. Physiotherapy treatment alone is unlikely to halt a rapidly progressive scoliosis during a growth spurt.

correction would cause a complication post-surgery. Bracing did not result in any complications; however, the curvature increased in this first brace with minor correction. Later, he was fitted with a Gensingen brace with a pronounced shift and a reasonable in-brace correction without any complications.

Using the current CAD/CAM standard, small children can also receive brace treatment. Younger patients with symptomatic scoliosis and/or syndromic scoliosis experience corrective results and comparatively few problems or difficulties with acclimatization. Fig. 8.29 shows a boy with a severe deformity in conjunction with neurofibromatosis who tolerated the CAD/CAM Chêneau- Gensingen® brace extremely well.

As with idiopathic scoliosis, symptomatic scoliosis and/or syndromic scoliosis also needs to be treated specifically, i.e., precisely according to its pattern, both during physiotherapy and brace treatment. At the conclusion of treatment, the x-ray image appears to be much less critical than a sound, cosmetically inconspicuous torso silhouette (Fig. 8.30). There is an art to selecting the appropriate therapeutic method to achieve this result (Weiss and Moramarco 2013a).

Findings-oriented physiotherapy for scoliosis uses the same corrective principles as pattern-oriented brace treatment. These corrective principles have been derived from decades of experience in physiotherapeutic treatment, a variety of experimentation with the various corrective options, and foremost, as a result of studying tens of thousands of x-ray examinations taken over the course of brace treatment and evaluating the corrective effects.

For this reason, the 'Best Practice' program described and the specific brace treatment corresponding to the individual curvature pattern in accordance with the 'Best Practice' standard (Gensingen brace) is regarded as the most up-to-date, evidence-based development and backed by a wealth of clinical experience.

Conservative scoliosis treatment, according to the Schroth 'Best Practice' standard, is a time-saving, simple, and, most-importantly, effective treatment approach that enjoys outstanding acceptance by patients (Weiss and Seibel 2010, Borysov and Borysov 2012, Pugacheva 2012, Lee 2014).

During a growth spurt, however, bracing must be regarded as the primary mode of treatment. The practitioner must be cognizant that physiotherapy alone is unlikely to halt a rapidly progressive scoliosis during a growth spurt (Fig. 8.31).

References

Appelgren G, Willner S. End Vertebra Angle – A Roentgenographic Method to Describe a Scoliosis. A Follow-up Study of Idiopathic Scoliosis Treated with the Boston Brace. Spine. 1990;15:71–74.

Asher MA, Burton DC. Adolescent idiopathic scoliosis: natural history and long-term treatment effects. Scoliosis. 2006;1(1):2.

Bettany-Saltikov J, Weiss HR, Chockalingam N, Taranu R, Srinivas S, Hogg J, Whittaker V, Kalyan RV. Surgical versus non-surgical interventions in patients with adolescent idiopathic scoliosis. Cochrane Protocol 2013.

Borysov M, Borysov A. Scoliosis short-term rehabilitation (SSTR) according to 'Best Practice' standards – are the results repeatable? Scoliosis. 2012 Jan 17;7(1):1.

Cheuk DKL, Wong V, Wraige E, Baxter P, Cole A. Cochrane Review (Group): Surgery for scoliosis in Duchenne muscular dystrophy. OA Musculoskeletal Medicine 2014 Apr 10;2(1):7.

Danielsson AJ, Hasserius R, Ohlin A, Nachemson AL. A prospective study of brace treatment versus observation alone in adolescent idiopathic scoliosis: a followup mean of 16 years after maturity. Spine. 2007 Sep 15;32(20):2198–2207.

Hopf C, Heine J. [Long-term results of the conservative treatment of scoliosis using the Cheneau brace]. Z Orthop Ihre Grenzgeb. 1985 May-Jun;123(3):312–322.

Landauer F, Wimmer C, Behensky H. Estimating the final outcome of brace treatment for idiopathic thoracic scoliosis at 6-month followup. Pediatr Rehabil. 2003;6(3–4):201–207.

Lee SG. Improvement of curvature and deformity in a sample of patients with Idiopathic Scoliosis with specific exercises. OA Musculoskeletal Medicine. 2014; Mar 12;2(1):6.

Negrini S, Minozzi S, Bettany-Saltikov J, Zaina F, Chockalingam N, Grivas TB, Kotwicki T, Maruyama T, Romano M, Vasiliadis ES. Braces for idiopathic scoliosis in adolescents. Cochrane Database Syst Rev. 2010 Jan 20;(1):CD006850.

Pugacheva N. Corrective exercises in multimodality therapy of idiopathic scoliosis in children - analysis of six weeks efficiency - pilot study. Stud Health Technol Inform. 2012; 176:365-371.

van Loon PJ, Kühbauch BA, Thunnissen FB. Forced lordosis on the thoracolumbar junction can correct coronal plane deformity in adolescents with double major curve pattern idiopathic scoliosis. Spine. 2008 Apr 1;33(7):797–801.

Weinstein SL, Dolan LA, Spratt KF, Peterson KK, Spoonamore MJ, Ponseti IV. Health and function of patients with untreated idiopathic scoliosis: A 50 Year Natural History Study. JAMA 2003;289(5):559–567.

Weinstein SL, Dolan LA, Wright JG, Dobbs MB. Effects of bracing in adolescents with idiopathic scoliosis. N Engl J Med. 2013;369:1512–1521.

Weiss HR, Rigo M, Chêneau J. Praxis der Chêneau-Korsettversorgung in der Skoliosetherapie. Georg Thieme Verlag, Stuttgart, 2000.

266

Weiss HR: Das "Sagittal Realignment Brace" (physio-logic® brace) in der Behandlung von erwachsenen Skoliosepatienten mit chronifiziertem Rückenschmerz. MOT 2005; 125:45–54.

Weiss HR. Differential indikation der Rumpforthesen in der Skoliosebehandlung, MOT , 2007;127: 66–70.

Weiss HR, Seibel S. Scoliosis short-term rehabilitation (SSTR) - a pilot investigation. The Internet Journal of Rehabilitation 2010; 1 Number 1.

Weiss HR. Korsettversorgung bei Skoliose Orthopädie Technik 62: 7. 488-498 July, 2011.

Weiss HR, Werkmann M. Rate of surgery in a sample of patients fulfilling the SRS inclusion criteria treated with a Chêneau brace of actual standard. Stud Health Technol Inform. 2012;176:407–410.

Weiss HR. Brace treatment in infantile/juvenile patients with progressive scoliosis is worthwhile. Stud Health Technol Inform. 2012, 176:383-386.

Weiss HR. History of soft brace treatment in patients with scoliosis: a critical appraisal. Hard Tissue. 2013 Jul 01;2(4):35.

Weiss HR, Moramarco M. Remodeling of trunk and back-shape deformities in patients with scoliosis using standardized asymmetric computer-aided design/computer-aided manufacturing braces. Hard Tissue. 2013a Feb 26;2(2):14.

Weiss HR, Moramarco M. Scoliosis-treatment indications according to current evidence. OA Musculoskeletal Medicine. 2013b Mar 01;1(1):1.

Weiss HR, Seibel S. Region of Interest in the radiological followup of patients with scoliosis. Hard Tissue. 2013 Jun 01;2(4):33.

Winter RB. Classification and terminology In: Lonstein J, Bradford   D, Winter R, Ogilvie J, editors. Moe's textbook of scoliosis and other spinal deformities. Philadelphia: WB Saunders 1995 p39-44.

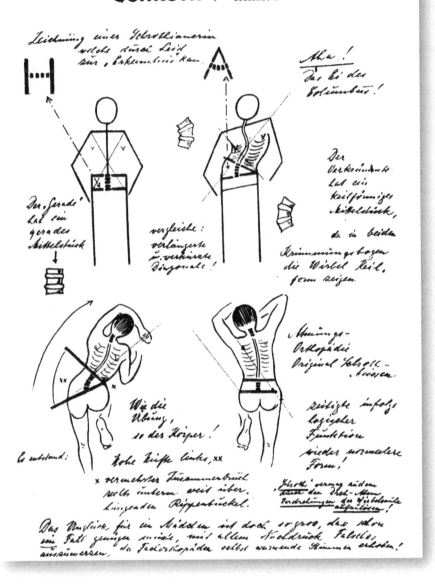

ORIGINAL-ATMUNGS-ORTHOPÄDIE
SCHROTH / MEISSEN, BOSELWEG 32

Original manuscript by Katharina Schroth

The Augmented Lehnert-Schroth (ALS) classification:

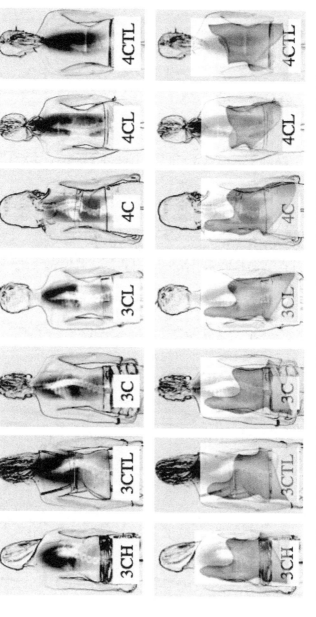

From left to right: 3CH (3-curve with hip prominence), 3CTL (3-curve with hip prominence thoracolumbar), 3C (3-curve balanced), 3CL (3-curve with long lumbar countercurve), 4C (4-curve double), 4CL (4-curve single lumbar) and 4CTL (4-curve single thoracolumbar).

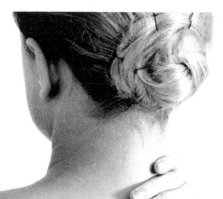
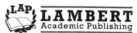

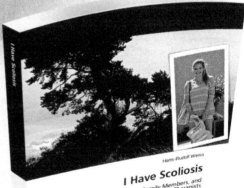
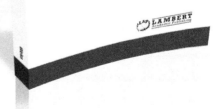

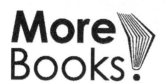
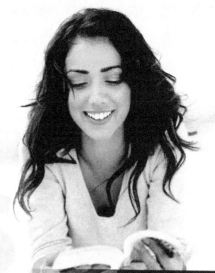

34410296R00159

Made in the USA
Middletown, DE
26 January 2019